O P L
OXFORD PSYCHIATRY LIBRARY

Obsessive-Compulsive Disorder

D0912784

O P L

OXFORD PSYCHIATRY LIBRARY

Obsessive-Compulsive Disorder

Prof. Dan J. Stein

Professor, Department of Psychiatry,
University of Cape Town, and
Director, Medical Research Council Unit on
Anxiety Disorders, South Africa

Prof. Naomi A. Fineberg

Consultant Psychiatrist at the National Obsessive
Compulsive Disorders Treatment Service, Queen
Elizabeth II Hospital, Welwyn Garden City, UK and
Visiting Professor, Postgraduate School of Medicine,
University of Hertfordshire, UK

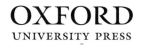

OXFORD
UNIVERSITY PRESS

OXFORD
UNIVERSITY PRESS

Great Clarendon Street, Oxford OX2 6DP

Oxford University Press is a department of the University of Oxford.
It furthers the University's objective of excellence in research, scholarship,
and education by publishing worldwide in

Oxford New York

Auckland Cape Town Dar es Salaam Hong Kong Karachi
Kuala Lumpur Madrid Melbourne Mexico City Nairobi
New Delhi Shanghai Taipei Toronto

With offices in

Argentina Austria Brazil Chile Czech Republic France Greece
Guatemala Hungary Italy Japan Poland Portugal Singapore
South Korea Switzerland Thailand Turkey Ukraine Vietnam

Oxford is a registered trade mark of Oxford University Press
in the UK and in certain other countries

Published in the United States
by Oxford University Press Inc., New York

British Library Cataloguing in Publication Data
Data available

Library of Congress Cataloging in Publication Data
Data available

Typeset by Newgen Imaging Systems (P) Ltd., Chennai, India
Printed in Italy
on acid-free paper by
LegoPrint S.p.A

ISBN 978–0–19–920460–1

10 9 8 7 6 5 4 3 2 1

Whilst every effort has been made to ensure that the contents of this book are as
complete, accurate and-up-to-date as possible at the date of writing. Oxford
University Press is not able to give any guarantee or assurance that such is the case.
Readers are urged to take appropriately qualified medical advice in all cases. The
information in this book is intended to be useful to the general reader, but should
not be used as a means of self-diagnosis or for the prescription of medication.

Contents

Chapter 1

Introduction

There are several reasons for thinking that obsessive-compulsive disorder (OCD) is one of the most important conditions in psychiatry.

First, epidemiological evidence has indicated that OCD may be one of the most prevalent and disabling of the psychiatric disorders (Karno et al 1988). Indeed, it is remarkable to note that in early data from a seminal WHO study of the burden of disease, OCD was characterized as one of the most disabling of all medical disorders (Murray & Lopez 1996). Although there remains some debate about the exact prevalence of OCD, there is no question that this condition is extremely costly, not only in terms of individual and family suffering (Amir et al 2000), but also in terms of cost to society (Hollander et al 1997). A consideration of the obsessive-compulsive disorders (OCDs), rather than just OCD, further expands the magnitude of the problem.

Second, OCD arguably comprises a paradigmatic exemplar of a neuropsychiatric disorder. It is a relatively homogeneous disorder, with studies consistently revealing an association with particular neurocircuitry (cortico-striatal-thalamic-cortical) and specific neurotransmitter systems (e.g. serotonin) (Stein 2002). Recent advances include molecular imaging studies of specific receptors in OCD, the demonstration that certain gene variants can play a causal role, and proof-of-principle studies that deep brain stimulation can rapidly reverse symptoms. Related mechanisms in the OCDs are being discovered. Although there may be important environmental contributors to OCD, the early view of OCD as caused by psychogenic conflict can no longer be supported (Stein & Stone 1997).

Third, OCD and OCDs provide physician-researchers and others interested in translational research with a unique opportunity to develop an integrated cognitive-affective neuroscience approach to psychiatric disorder. OCD was not only one of the first disorders shown in controlled studies to respond to both pharmacotherapy and psychotherapy, it was the first condition in which both treatment modalities were demonstrated to normalize the underlying functional neuroanatomy. The growing set of animal, genetic, and molecular imaging studies of OCD, taken together with rigorous work on the phenomenology and neurocircuitry of OCD and OCDs, provide a unique opportunity for scientists to develop translation models of obsessive-compulsive psychopathology, and to move between bench and bedside in studying its treatment.

Fourth, there is now an extensive database of randomized controlled trials of treatment of OCD, allowing for an evidence-based approach to its management. This database covers both pharmacotherapy and psychotherapy, both first-line and augmentation trials, both acute and long-term studies, and studies in both adults and children (Fineberg & Gale, 2005). Professional organizations have drawn on this extensive database in order to develop high-quality guidelines and algorithms for the treatment of OCD. Consumer organizations have been able to encourage people suffering from OCD symptoms to establish an early diagnosis and to receive appropriate treatment. Although additional work is needed to move the investigation of OCD from studies of efficacy to those of effectiveness in real-world settings, there is already an important opportunity to take knowledge from randomized controlled trials and to apply it in every-day practice. The database on OCDs is smaller, but similarly has a great deal of clinical utility.

This volume will summarize the phenomenology, pathogenesis, pharmacotherapy and psychotherapy of OCD. Many reviews exist in the academic literature of each of these areas. The aim of the current volume is to synthesize the findings in a succinct and practical way, in order that it is as useful as possible for clinicians, and hopefully, therefore, also for patients suffering from OCD.

References

Amir, N., Freshman, M., Foa, E.B. (2000). Family distress and involvement in relatives of obsessive-compulsive disorder patients. *J. Anxiety Disord.*, **14**: 209–217.

Fineberg, N.A., Gale, T.M. (2005). Evidence-based pharmacotherapy of obsessive-compulsive disorder. *Int. J. Neuropsychopharmacol.*, **8**: 107–129.

Hollander, E., Stein, D.J., Broatch, J., Himelein, C., Rowland, C. (1997). A pharmacoeconomic and quality of life study of obsessive-compulsive disorder. *CNS Spectrums*, **2**: 16–25.

Karno, M., Goldin, J.M., Sorenson, S.B., et al. (1988). The epidemiology of obsessive-compulsive disorder in five US communities. *Archs Gen. Psychiat.*, **45**: 1094–1099.

Murray, C.J.L., Lopez, A.D. (1996). *Global Burden of Disease: A Comprehensive Assessment of Mortality and Morbidity from Diseases, Injuries and Risk Factors in 1990 and Projected to 2020*, Vol. I. Harvard, World Health Organization.

Stein, D.J. (2002). Seminar on obsessive-compulsive disorder. *Lancet*, **360**: 397–405.

Stein, D.J., Stone, M.H. (1997). *Essential Papers on Obsessive-Compulsive Disorders*. New York University Press, New York.

Chapter 2

Phenomenology

Key points

- OCD is a common lifespan illness that causes substantial suffering
- Patients tend to hide symptoms and OCD is frequently overlooked by health professionals
- Factor analyses consistently identify particular symptom clusters in OCD
- Direct enquiry about OCD can help accurately identify the illness
- Measures for screening, diagnosis, and assessing OCD symptom severity are available

2.1 Symptoms

OCD is characterized by intrusive, unpleasant thoughts or images (obsessions), and by repetitive, unwanted actions (compulsions) that are performed in response to obsessions or according to rigid rules. Although obsessions increase anxiety, they are not simply real-life worries. The consequent compulsions may serve to decrease or increase anxiety. The diagnostic criteria for OCD in the *Diagnostic and Statistical Manual of Mental Disorders* (DSM-IV-TR) (American Psychiatric Association 2000) emphasize that compulsions can be either observable behaviours or mental rituals. While patients typically recognize the excessiveness of their symptoms, there is a range of insight and some may be classified as suffering from the 'poor insight' subtype (Box 2.1).

A broad range of possible obsessions and compulsions may be found. The most common involve concerns about contamination with consequent washing, or concerns about harm to self or others with consequent checking. Factor analysis has demonstrated additional subgroups involving symptom clusters such as symmetry concerns and arranging rituals, hoarding and collecting (Leckman et al 2001) (Box 2.2). Other common symptoms include sexual, religious, somatic, and musical obsessions (Stein et al 2001).

While predominant symptoms may alter for an individual over time (Swedo et al 1989), the constancy of OCD symptomatology across time (pathological scrupulosity, for example) and place (similar symptoms occur across many cultures) is striking (Stein & Rapoport 1996). Moreover, symptoms in children and adults appear remarkably similar, although they may reflect the developmental level; for example, young children may have more concrete kinds of rituals.

Symptoms differ to some degree in patients with and without tics (Miguel et al 2001), perhaps pointing to underlying biological differences (see Chapter 3). Patients with obsessional slowness may also have another form of OCD that is characterized by a greater degree of neurological impairment (Veale 1993).

Box 2.1 DSM-IV diagnostic criteria for OCD

A. Either obsessions or compulsions:

Obsessions as defined by (1), (2), (3) and (4):

(1) recurrent and persistent thoughts, impulses, or images that are experienced, at some time during the disturbance, as intrusive and inappropriate and that cause marked anxiety or distress

(2) the thoughts, impulses, or images are not simply excessive worries about real-life problems

(3) the person attempts to ignore or suppress such thoughts, impulses, or images, or to neutralize them with some other thought or action

(4) the person recognizes that the obsessional thoughts, impulses, or images are a product of his or her own mind (not imposed from without as in thought insertion)

Compulsions as defined by (1) and (2):

(1) repetitive behaviours (e.g. hand washing, ordering, checking) or mental acts (e.g. praying, counting, repeating words silently) that the person feels driven to perform in response to an obsession, or according to rules that must be applied rigidly

(2) the behaviours or mental acts are aimed at preventing or reducing distress or preventing some dreaded event or situation; however, these behaviours or mental acts either are not connected in a realistic way with what they are designed to neutralize or prevent or are clearly excessive.

B. At some point during the course of the disorder, the person has recognized that the obsessions or compulsions are excessive or unreasonable. Note: This does not apply to children.

C. The obsessions or compulsions cause marked distress, are time consuming (take more than 1hr per day), or significantly interfere with the person's normal routine, occupational (or academic) functioning, or usual social activities or relationships.

D. If another Axis I disorder is present, the content of the obsessions or compulsions is not restricted to it (e.g. preoccupation with food in the presence of an eating disorder; hair pulling in the presence of trichotillomania; concern with appearance in the presence of body dysmorphic disorder; preoccupation with drugs in the presence of a substance use disorder; preoccupation with having a serious illness in the presence of hypochondriasis; preoccupation with sexual urges or fantasies in the presence of a paraphilia; or guilty ruminations in the presence of major depressive disorder).

E. The disturbance is not due to the direct physiological effects of a substance (e.g. a drug of abuse, a medication) or a general medical condition.

Specify if:

With poor insight: if, for most of the time during the current episode, the person does not recognize that the obsessions and compulsions are excessive or unreasonable.

Box 2.2 **OCD symptom clusters**	
Obsessions	**Compulsions**
Contamination concerns	Washing, bathing, showering
Harm to self/others, sexual/religious concerns	Checking, praying, asking for reassurance
Symmetry, precision concerns	Arranging, ordering
Saving concerns	Hoarding

2.2 Diagnostic threshold

By definition, OCD symptoms are accompanied by marked distress and dysfunction; this is the standard clinical significance criterion in DSM-IV-TR (Spitzer & Wakefield 1999). Subclinical obsessive-compulsive symptoms may be fairly common, and are certainly seen during the course of normal development. In patients with OCD, however, it is usually not difficult to appreciate the tremendous suffering associated with this condition. Indeed, a number of recent studies have documented that quality of life in OCD is severely affected (Stein *et al* 2000).

2.3 Differential diagnosis

The DSM-IV-TR criteria for OCD indicate that symptoms should not be due to a general medical disorder nor to a substance. As discussed in more detail below, obsessive-compulsive symptoms may be seen in a range of neurological lesions involving cortico-striatal-thalamic-cortical (CSTC) circuits; they may emerge after the administration of dopamine agonists (such as methylphenidate or cocaine); or they may emerge in the context of streptococcal infection (presumably on an auto-immune basis).

Although the distinction between Axis I and II disorders is blurred at times, the obsessions and compulsions of OCD should not be confused with the inflexible character traits that constitute obsessive-compulsive personality disorder such as perfectionism and overconscientiousness. Similarly, despite occasional overlap, OCD symptoms differ clearly from the fears and worries seen in other anxiety disorders, from the ruminations characteristic of mood disorders, and from the delusions of psychotic disorders.

Obsessive-compulsive symptoms comprise an intrinsic component of a number of neuropsychiatric conditions, including autism, Tourette's syndrome, and frontal lobe lesions. Conversely, other disorders entail a restricted focus on specific symptoms that can also be seen in OCD, for example, body dysmorphic disorder (concerns about imagined ugliness) and hypochondriasis (concerns about imagined illness), both involve somatic obsessions and compulsions. Eating disorders such as anorexia nervosa involve obsessive preoccupation with body size and shape and eating patterns. Indeed, it has been suggested that disorders with overlapping phenomenology and psychobiology with OCD fall within a putative spectrum of obsessive-compulsive disorders (OCDs) (Hollander 1993). The boundaries and underpinnings of this construct remain to be elucidated.

2.4 **Prevalence**

The Epidemiological Catchment Area (ECA) studies provided the first epidemiological data on OCD that were based on a nationally representative sample and reliable diagnostic criteria. OCD was found to be the fourth most prevalent psychiatric disorder, with a lifetime prevalence of 2.5% (Karno et al 1988). A cross-national study employing similar methodology demonstrated similar prevalence rates across a range of different populations (Weissman et al 1994). A review of community studies suggested that despite some concerns about the validity of the diagnosis of OCD in the ECA studies (Nelson & Rice 1997), OCD is common in both adult (Bebbington et al 1998) and paediatric (Zohar 1999) populations, with many studies yielding a prevalence similar to that found by the ECA investigators (Wittchen & Jacobi 2005; Kessler et al 2006).

The male to female ratio of OCD is roughly similar, in contrast to many other anxiety and mood disorders, in which the prevalence in females is higher. Age of onset in OCD may have a bimodal distribution. A subset of patients has onset at puberty or earlier; juvenile-onset OCD may be particularly common in males, and appears to have other distinguishing characteristics such as greater familiality and relationship to tic disorders (Eichstedt & Arnold 2001). Patients with a later onset include those developing OCD after pregnancy, miscarriage, or parturition (Geller et al 2001; Williams & Koran 1997).

2.5 **Comorbidity**

Epidemiological studies are consistent with clinical work showing a substantial lifetime comorbidity with other mental disorders including depression, which developed in approximately two thirds of cases presenting for treatment, specific phobia (22%), social phobia (18%), eating disorder (17%), alcohol dependence (14%), panic disorder (12%) and Tourette's syndrome (7%) (Pigott et al 1994). They also suggested that a subgroup of OCD patients may have impulsive features, including childhood conduct disorder symptoms, attentional deficits and an increased rate of suicide attempts (Hollander et al 1997).

2.6 **Course and burden of illness**

Although acute episodes of OCD have been documented (Ravizza et al 1996), and considerable variability exists in the periodicity, duration, and severity of illness, OCD is usually a chronic disorder (Pinto *et al* 2006). Complete recovery is not commonly reported (Skoog & Skoog 1999), but cases are likely to show improvements over time (Angst *et al* 2004). Intermittent episodes of OCD are thought to occur more frequently in the early stages of illness, and those with an early episodic course may experience a better long-term prognosis (Skoog & Skoog 1999).

OCD is associated with significant direct and indirect costs (Dupont *et al* 1995). These are compounded by a lack of recognition, under-diagnosis, and inappropriate treatment. Patients may be too embarrassed to visit a clinician, or may not be aware that help is available; the lag time from symptom onset to correct diagnosis was 17 years in one survey (Hollander *et al* 1997). The World Health Organization recently ranked OCD within the twenty leading causes of medical disability. In view of the substantial socio-economic costs associated with untreated OCD, estimated in one American study as 6% of the total cost associated with mental illness (Dupont *et al* 1995) and the development of cost-effective therapies that can be offered in primary or secondary medical care settings, better recognition and treatment of the disorder is now starting to be recognized by government health departments as a major public health objective (e.g. www.nice.org.uk).

2.7 OCD in the non-psychiatric setting

Given that patients often conceal their symptoms (Newth & Rachman 2001), it is important to be aware of the possible presentation of OCD in a range of psychiatric and non-psychiatric medical settings. In dermatology clinics, for example, washing rituals may be common. Patients asking for cosmetic surgery may suffer from somatic obsessions, patients in general medical clinics from hypochondriacal obsessions, neurology patients with involuntary movement disorders (Tourette's syndrome, Sydenham's chorea, Huntington's disorder) may have comorbid OCD, paediatric patients may have OCD after streptoccocal infection, and pregnant patients may experience de-novo or increased OCD symptoms either during pregnancy or after delivery. Box 2.3 shows just some of the common areas where OCD patients present for treatment.

2.8 Awareness and screening

Despite growing awareness, most doctors and nurses are not trained to detect OCD. Given patients' reluctance about disclosure, it is important for clinicians to ask the right questions. Although it can take years before individuals find a health professional in whom they can confide, direct enquiry by a sympathetic health practitioner is

Box 2.3 Presentations for treatment

Professional	Reason for consultation
GP	Depression, anxiety
Dermatologist	Chapped hands, eczema, trichotillomania,
Cosmetic surgeon	Concerns about appearance (body dysmorphic disorder)
Oncologist	Fear of cancer
Genito-urinary	Fear of HIV
Neurologist	OCD associated with Tourette's syndrome
Obstetrician	OCD during pregnancy or the puerperium
Gynaecologist	Vaginal discomfort from douching

Box 2.4 Zohar–Fineberg Obsessive Compulsive Screen (Z-FOCS): five screening questions for obsessive-compulsive disorder

1. Do you wash or clean a lot?
2. Do you check things a lot?
3. Is there any thought that keeps bothering you that you would like to get rid of but can't?
4. Do your daily activities take a long time to finish?
5. Are you concerned about orderliness or symmetry?

© Joseph Zohar and Naomi A. Fineberg, 2006.

usually successful. Arguably, practitioners in areas known to attract large numbers of patients need to be primed to look for characteristic symptoms and enquire proactively, using targeted questions. Mental health workers should consider incorporating a form of 'brief screening' into every mental state examination (Heyman et al 2006).

The Zohar–Fineberg Obsessive Compulsive Screen (Z-FOCS) (Box 2.4) was devised by J. Zohar for the International Council on OCD. It consists of five simple questions designed to be administered by a doctor or a nurse and takes less than one minute to administer (Fineberg & Roberts 2001). A positive response to any of the questions should lead to detailed enquiry for OCD.

2.9 Assessment

Evaluation of OCD requires a thorough psychiatric history and examination to assess OCD symptoms and comorbid disorders, and to allow a differential diagnosis from other anxiety, mood, and psychotic disorders. A general medical history and examination should also be obtained. In some patients, OCD symptoms begin in the aftermath of infection (Swedo et al 1998). Comorbid tics are not uncommon but are often overlooked and patients should be carefully observed for them as they may signal a different treatment pathway. Similarly children with OCD should be asked about problems with attention and concentration since ADHD may easily be missed. Indications for special investigations such as structural brain imaging might include late onset, atypical symptoms, or severe treatment refractoriness.

Although the diagnosis is usually confirmed by a clinical interview, the use of brief standardized interviews, such as the Mini International Neuropsychiatric Interview (MINI) (Sheehan et al 1994) for diagnosis may be useful. It may also be helpful to inquire about the patient's own explanatory model of their disorder – their theories of its cause and treatment. Patients with scrupulosity, for example, may see their symptoms in religious terms (Ciarrochi 1995). Some patients adhere to a view that unresolved, unconscious conflict is a cause of symptoms, others that lack of self-confidence or fears of losing control are responsible. Being aware of these models, and offering alternative perspectives, are key steps in starting treatment. Consumer advocacy groups (Stein et al 2001) and internet virtual groups (Stein 1997) may usefully contribute to such psycho-education (see Chapter 6).

People with OCD are notoriously poor at gauging their level of impairment, particularly during treatment when they may have difficulty recognizing signs of improvement. It can be helpful to ask a family member to corroborate the patient's history. The Yale–Brown Obsessive Compulsive Scale (Y-BOCS) (Goodman et al 1989) measures the severity of OCD. It is sufficiently user-friendly to be easily administered in clinical practice, and its reliability and validity and sensitivity to change have made it the current 'gold standard' in OCD randomized controlled trials. The scale has also been adapted for use in children and adolescents (Appendix I, II: Y-BOCS, CY-BOCS), and for assessment of OCD spectrum disorders such as dysmorphic disorder. The Dimensional Y-BOCS extends the Y-BOCS to allow evaluation of OCD-severity according to current dimensional models of OCD and symptom clusters (Appendix: DY-BOCS). The Clinical Global ImpressionSeverity and -Improvement Scales (Guy 1976) are rapid measures of global severity and improvement that have been well validated for OCD and shown to be sensitive to change in treatment trials.

References

American Psychiatric Association (1994). *Diagnostic and Statistical Manual of Mental Disorders*, 4th edn. American Psychiatric Press, Washington, DC.

Angst, J., Gamma, A., Endrass, J., et al. (2004). Obsessive-compulsive severity spectrum in the community: prevalence, comorbidity, and course. *Eur. Archs Psychiat., Clin. Neurosci.,* **254**(3): 156–164.

Bebbington, P.E. (1998). Epidemiology of obsessive-compulsive disorder. *Br. J. Psychiat.,* Suppl **35**: 2–6.

Ciarrocchi, J.W. (1995). *The Doubting Disease: Help for Scrupulosity and Religious Compulsions.* Paulist Press, Mahwah, NJ.

Dupont, R.L., Rice, D.P., Shiraki, S., et al. (1995). Economic costs of obsessive-compulsive disorder. *Med. Interface,* **8**: 102–109.

Eichstedt, J.A., Arnold, S.L. (2001). Childhood-onset obsessive-compulsive disorder: a tic-related subtype of OCD? *Clin. Psychol. Rev.,* **21**: 137–157.

Fineberg, N.A., Roberts, A. (2001). Obsessive compulsive disorder: a twenty-first century perspective. In Fineberg, N.A., Marazitti, D., Stein, D. eds, *Obsessive Compulsive Disorder: A Practical Guide.* Martin Dunitz, London.

Geller, P.A., Klier, C.M., Neugebauer, R. (2001). Anxiety disorders following miscarriage. *J. Clin. Psychiat.,* **62**: 432–438.

Goodman, W.K., Price, L.H., Rasmussen, S.A., et al. (1989). The Yale-Brown Obsessive Compulsive Scale. I. Development, use, and reliability. *Archs Gen. Psychiat.,* **46**: 1006–1011.

Guy W. (1976) ECDEU Assessment Manual for Psychopharmacology, revised. US Dept Health, Education, and Welfare publication (ADM) 76–338. Rockville, MD, National Institute of Mental Health.

Heyman I, Mataix-Cols D, Fineberg NA. Obsessive-compulsive disorder. *Brit Medical J,* **333**: 26th August 2006, 424–429.

Hollander, E. (1993). *Obsessive-Compulsive Related Disorders.* American Psychiatric Press, Washington, DC.

Hollander, E., Greenwald, S., Neville, D., et al. (1997). Uncomplicated and comorbid obsessive-compulsive disorder in an epidemiologic sample. *Depress. Anxiety,* **4**: 111–119.

Hollander, E., Stein, D.J., Broatch, et al. (1997). A pharmacoeconomic and quality of life study of obsessive-compulsive disorder. *CNS Spectrums,* **2**: 16–25.

Karno, M., Goldin, J.M., Sorenson, S.B., et al. (1988). The epidemiology of obsessive compulsive disorder in five US communities. *Archs Gen. Psychiat.,* **45**: 1094–1099.

Kessler R.C., Berglund P., Demler D., et al. (2005). Lifetime prevalence and age of onset distribution of DSM-IV disorders in the National Comorbidity Survey Replication. *Arch Gen Psychiatry,* **62**: 593–602.

Leckman, J.F., Zhang, H., Alsobrook, J.P., et al. (2001). Symptom dimensions in obsessive-compulsive disorder: toward quantitative phenotypes. *Am. J. Med. Genet.,* **105**: 28–30.

Miguel, E.C., do Rosario-Campos, M.C., Shavitt, R.G., Hounie, A.G., et al. (2001). The tic-related obsessive-compulsive disorder phenotype and treatment implications. *Adv. Neurol.,* **85**: 43–55.

Nelson, E., Rice, J. (1997). Stability of diagnosis of obsessive-compulsive disorder in the Epidemiologic Catchment Area study. *Am. J. Psychiat.,* **154**: 826–831.

Newth, S., Rachman, S. (2001). The concealment of obsessions. *Behav. Res. Ther.,* **39**: 457–464.

Pigott T.A., L'Heureux, F., Dubbert, B., et al. (1994). Obsessive compulsive disorder: comorbid conditions. *J. Clin. Psychiat.*, **55**(Suppl): 15–27; discussion 28–32. Review.

Pinto A., Mancebo M.C., Eisen J.L., et al. The Brown Longitudinal Obsessive Compulsive Study: clinical features and symptoms of the sample at intake. *J Clin Psychiatry* 2006 May; **67(5)**: 703–11.

Ravizza, L, Barzega, G., Bellino, S., et al. (1996). Drug treatment of obsessive–compulsive disorder (OCD): Long-term trial with clomipramine and selective serotonin reuptake inhibitors (SSRIs). *Psychopharmacol. Bull.*, **32**: 167–173.

Sheehan, D.V., Lecrubier, Y., Janavs, J., et al. (1994). *Mini International Neuropsychiatric Interview* (MINI). Tampa, University of South Florida Institute for Research in Psychiatry, Florida, and INSERM – Hôpital de la Salpetrière, Paris.

Spitzer, R.L. and Wakefield, J.C. (1999). DSM-IV diagnostic criterion for clinical significance: Does it help solve the false positive problem? *Am. J. Psychiat.*, **156**: 1856–1864.

Skoog, G., Skoog, I. (1999). A 40-year follow-up of patients with obsessive-compulsive disorder. *Archs Gen. Psychiat.*, **56**: 121–127.

Stein, D.J, Fineberg, N, Harvey, B. (2001). Unusual symptoms of OCD. In Fineberg, N., Marazziti, D. Stein, D.J. eds, *Obsessive Compulsive Disorder: A Practical Guide.* Martin Dunitz, London, 37–50.

Stein, D.J. (1997). Psychiatry on the internet: survey of an OCD mailing list. *Psychiat. Bull.*, **21**: 95–98.

Stein, D.J., Allen, A., Bobes, J., et al. (2000). Quality of life in obsessive-compulsive disorder. *CNS Spectrums*, **5**(Suppl 4): 37–39.

Stein, D.J., Rapoport, J. L. (1996). Cross-cultural studies and obsessive-compulsive disorder. *CNS Spectrums*, **1**: 42–46.

Stein, D.J., Wessels, C., Zungu-Dirwayi, N., Berk, M., Wilson, Z. (2001). Value and effectiveness of consumer advocacy groups: a survey of the anxiety disorders support group in South Africa. *Depressn Anxiety*, **13**: 105–107.

Swedo, S.E., Leonard, H.L., Garvey, M., et al. (1998). Pediatric autoimmune neuropsychiatric disorders associated with streptococcal infections: clinical description of the first 50 cases. *Am. J. Psychiat.*, **155**: 264–271.

Swedo, S., Schapiro, M.G., Grady, C.L., et al. (1989). Cerebral glucose metabolism in childhood onset obsessive-compulsive disorder. *Archs Gen. Psychiat.* **46**: 518–523.

Veale, D. (1993). Classification and treatment of obsessional slowness. *Br. J. Psychiat.*, **162**: 198–203.

Weissman, M.M., Bland, R.C., Canino, G.J., et al. (1994). The cross national epidemiology of obsessive compulsive disorder. *J. Clin. Psychiat.*, **55**(Suppl): 5–10.

Williams, K.E. and Koran, L.M. (1997). Obsessive-compulsive disorder in pregnancy, the puerperium, and the premenstruum. *J. Clin. Psychiat.*, **58**: 330–334.

Wittchen H.U., Jacobi F. Size and burden of mental disorder in Europe: a critical review and appraisal of 27 studies. *Eur Neuropsychopharmacol 2005*; **15**: 357–76.

Zohar, A.H. (1999). The epidemiology of obsessive-compulsive disorder in children and adolescents. *Child Adolesc. Psychiat. Clin. North Am.* **8**: 445–460.

Chapter 3

Pathogenesis

Key points

- Cortico-striatal-thalamic-cortical (CSTC) neurocircuitry plays a key role in OCD
- Serotonin (5-HT) and dopamine (DA) receptors in CSTC circuits appear particularly important
- Particular variations in 5-HT and DA genes may contribute to vulnerability to OCD
- Immune mechanisms may also play a role in contributing to CTSC dysfunction
- OCD may involve a failure to inhibit evolutionarily-based procedural strategies
- Both pharmacotherapy (SSRIs) and psychotherapy (CBT) can reverse CSTC dysfunction

3.1 Introduction

In this chapter we review current understanding of the pathogenesis of OCD. Whereas OCD was once primarily conceptualized as a psychogenic disorder, it is now increasingly conceptualized as a neuropsychiatric condition, mediated by a specific neurocircuitry. As we understand more about the cognitive and affective phenomena mediated by the neuronal abnormalities in this disorder, and as we learn about the genes and proteins which mediate these neuronal changes, so an integrated cognitive-affective neuroscience of OCD becomes possible.

3.2 Neuroanatomy

Perhaps the earliest indication that OCD is mediated by specific neuronal circuits came from work showing an association between post-encephalitis parkinsonian and obsessive-compulsive symptoms together with striatal lesions (Cheyette & Cummings 1995). OCD symptoms in a range of neurological disorders with striatal involvement, including Tourette's syndrome, Sydenham's chorea, Huntington's disorder and Parkinson's disorder were also documented by early authors (Stein et al 1994) (see Table 3.1). Such findings have been confirmed in a range of more recent systematic investigations.

Table 3.1 **Lesions of the Basal Ganglia Associated with OCD (Stein, 2003)**	
Infectious/Immune	postencephalitic parkinsonism, Sydenham's chorea
Traumatic/Toxic	head injury, wasp sting, manganese intoxication
Vascular/Hypoxic	infarction, carbon monoxide intoxication, neonatal hypoxia
Genetic/Idiopathic	Tourette's syndrome, Huntington's disease, neuroacanthocytosis

Conversely, OCD patients have been found to demonstrate abnormalities in a broad series of measures and paradigms used in neuropsychiatric (e.g. neurological soft signs, olfactory identification, evoked potentials, prepulse inhibition, intracortical inhibition) and neuropsychological (e.g. executive function, visual memory function) research (Stein et al 1994; Purcell et al 1998a). These neuropsychiatric and neuropsychological abnormalities have consistently pointed to cortico-striatal-thalamo-cortical (CSTC) dysfunction and impaired control of behavioural inhibition, and some evidence has suggested that they are relatively specific to OCD (Purcell et al. 1998b).

Advances in brain imaging have, however, provided the most persuasive neuroanatomic data on OCD (Rauch & Baxter 1998; Whiteside et al 2004). Structural imaging has pointed, in a number of studies, to abnormalities such as decreased volume or increased gray matter density in CSTC circuits. Discrepancies in structural imaging studies may partly reflect the heterogeneity of OCD; for example, patients with OCD secondary to streptococcal infection (see below) may have increased striatal volumes (Giedd et al 2000), whereas patients with more chronic illness may have decreased volumes.

Functional imaging has consistently found that OCD is characterized by increased activity in orbitofrontal cortex, cingulate, and striatum at rest and especially during exposure to feared stimuli (Figure 3.1). Somewhat different circuits may be involved in mediating the different OCD symptom clusters (Saxena et al 2004; Mataix-Cols et al 2005). The use of sophisticated cognitive and affective paradigms has confirmed the involvement of CSTC circuits in OCD (Rauch et al 2001; Fitzgerald et al 2004; Remijnse et al 2006); for example during implicit learning OCD subjects do not show the expected increase in striatal activity, but instead employ more temporal cortical regions (Rauch et al 2001).

The application of molecular imaging methods to OCD is at an early stage (Rosenberg et al 2001; Benazon et al 2003; Denys et al 2004a; Talbot 2004; van der Wee et al 2004), but supports the structural and functional findings. Thus magnetic resonance spectroscopy (MRS) demonstrated alterations in various metabolites in

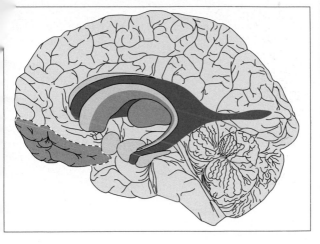

Figure 3.1 Increased activity in orbitofrontal cortex, ventral striatum, and thalamus in OCD. (Reproduced with permission of the University of Stellenbosch.)

CSTC circuits in OCD, while studies of dopaminergic receptors in the striatum have also demonstrated abnormalities.

Other regions of the brain have less commonly been suggested to play a role in OCD. For example, temporal dysfunction has occasionally been associated with OCD (Hugo et al 1999; Zungu-Dirwayi 1999), and there is some evidence of amygdala involvement (Szeszko et al 1999). Paediatric imaging research has supported the involvement of CTSC circuits in OCD, and potentially offers the promise of being able to determine the evolution of brain abnormalities in different regions over time (Rosenberg & Keshavan 1998).

Remarkably, both successful pharmacotherapy and behavioural therapy are able to normalize activity in CSTC circuits (Baxter et al 1992) (Figure 3.2). It is notable that OCD was the first disorder in which studies of this kind were done, and subsequent analogous work in other disorders has contributed to an integrated view of the mind–body. Interestingly, baseline activity differentially predicts response to pharmacotherapy and to psychotherapy (Brody et al 1998), so that different modalities may be effective via different mechanisms. Neurosurgical interruption of CSTC circuits may also reduce symptoms (Jenike 1998; Rauch et al 2004) and decrease striatal volume (Rauch 2000).

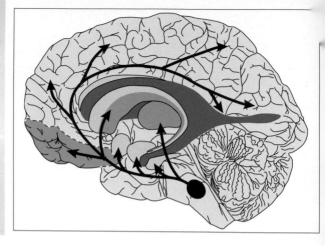

Figure 3.2 Normalization of cortico-striatal-thalamic-cortical (CSTC) circuits by either pharmacotherapy or psychotherapy in OCD. The black arrows represent the serotonergic neurons originating in the raphe, and projecting widely to CSTC and other regions. (Reproduced with permission of the University of Stellenbosch.)

3.3 **Neurochemistry**

A range of evidence points to the role of the serotonin (5-HT) system in mediating OCD. The earliest evidence for this came from reports that clomipramine, a tricyclic antidepressant that is predominantly a 5-HT reuptake inhibitor (SRI), was effective in the treatment of OCD (Fernandez-Cordoba & Lopez-Ibor Alino 1967). These early reports were subsequently confirmed by controlled trials comparing clomipramine with noradrenergic reuptake inhibitors (Zohar & Insel 1987), and with placebo (DeVeaugh-Geiss et al 1991). Clomipramine administration was shown to be accompanied by a decrease in cerebrospinal fluid concentrations of the 5-HT metabolite, 5-hydroxy-indoleacetic acid (CSF 5-HIAA) in OCD patients (Thoren et al 1980).

Studies of static measures of serotonergic function in OCD have, however, been somewhat inconsistent, and other work has focused on more informative dynamic measures (Baumgarten & Grozdanovic 1998). Thus, for example, administration of the 5-HT agonist m-chlorophenylpiperazine (mCPP) has been accompanied by exacerbation of OCD symptoms and a blunted neuroendocrine response in some (although not all) studies. Molecular imaging studies of the 5-HT system in OCD are at an early stage, but further progress can be expected as more serotonergic radioligands become available (Simpson et al 2003; Adams et al 2005). Notably, after treatment with an SRI, behavioural and neuroendocrine responses to mCPP appear normalized (Zohar et al 1988).

An immediate question is the possible role of specific 5-HT sub-receptors in OCD. Effects of mCPP on the postsynaptic $5-HT_{2C}$ receptor, for example, may be particularly relevant to understanding its action in OCD (Delgado & Moreno 1998; Bergqvist et al 1999). Preclinical data also suggest that the $5-HT_{1B}$ terminal autoreceptor plays an important role; its desensitization in orbitofrontal cortex requires high duration/dose administration of SRIs, reminiscent of clinical findings (see below) (El Mansari et al, 1995). Preliminary challenge (Koran et al 2001), pharmacological (Stern et al 1998), genetic (Mundo et al 2000) and imaging (Stein 1999) data support a role for $5-HT_{1B}$ in OCD.

Perhaps the most convincing evidence that serotonergic abnormalities can lead to OCD comes from genetic studies showing that, in a small percentage of OCD subjects, specific functional gene variants in the serotonin system are associated with OCD (Ozaki et al 2003). However, there is so far relatively little convincing evidence that any specific abnormality in the 5-HT system has an aetiological role in most patients. Indeed, a range of other systems, including glutamate neurotransmission (Carlsson 2001), certain neuropeptides (McDougle et al 1999), and gonadal steroids (Williams & Koran 1997; Lochner & Stein 2001) may also play a role. Ultimately the role of second and third messenger pathways in OCD will need to be delineated (Marazziti et al 2000; Perez et al 2000; Harvey et al 2001).

One CSTC neurotransmitter system that may be particularly important in mediating OCD in some patients is dopamine (Goodman et al 1990). In preclinical studies, administration of dopamine agonists leads to stereotypic behaviour, while in humans such agents may exacerbate OCD symptoms and tics (Denys et al 2006). Molecular imaging studies have documented altered binding in specific dopamine receptors in OCD (Denys et al 2004; van der Wee et al 2004). Conversely, dopamine blockers are used in the treatment of Tourette's syndrome, a putative OCD spectrum disorder. Furthermore, there is growing evidence (see below) that augmentation of SRIs with such agents may be useful in treatment-refractory OCD (Fineberg & Gale 2005; Ipser et al 2006).

3.4 Neurogenetics

Early work suggesting that OCD has a familial component has been confirmed by more recent rigorous studies that have used structured diagnostic interviews of probands and controls (Hettema et al 2001; van Grootheest et al 2005). Also, several studies have demonstrated a genetic relationship between OCD and Tourette's syndrome (Pauls & Alsobrook 1999). Patients with OCD symptoms and a family history of Tourette's may have neurobiological dysfunction more similar to Tourette's than to primary OCD (Moriarty et al 1997).

There is increasing interest in the possibility that functional genetic polymorphisms may play a role in the pathogenesis of OCD (Pato 2001; Hemmings & Stein 2006). Although not all studies are consistent there is accumulating evidence that polymorphisms in serotonergic genes (See Table 3.2), some dopaminergic genes, and catechol-O-methyltransferase (COMT) may all contribute to vulnerability to OCD (Hemmings et al 2002; Azzam & Mathews 2003; Hasler et al 2006) and some of its subtypes (Nicolini et al 1998; Hemmings et al 2004). There is also interesting preliminary data suggesting that variants in a range of other genes, including glutamate receptors, gamma-aminobutyric acid (GABA) receptors, opioid receptors, and neurotrophic genes may play a role in the disorder (Arnold et al 2004; Arnold et al 2006; Zai et al 2004, 2005; Urraca 2004).

A number of other approaches to determining the genetic basis of OCD may also yield important results. Animal models may be useful in suggesting a role for particular genes in stereotypic behaviour (Berridge et al 2005). Genetic findings in OCD spectrum disorders such as Tourette's may ultimately lead to an understanding of a range of related conditions (Abelson et al 2005; Zuchner 2006). Patients with obsessive-compulsive symptoms secondary to chromosomal deletions may provide intriguing clues about which genes are involved in mediating the disorder (Gothelf et al 2004). Whole genome scanning has similarly suggested that a number of chromosomal regions may be particularly important in OCD (Shugart et al 2006). Such work is exciting insofar as it may ultimately provide the basis for a rational approach to delineating the heterogeneity of OCD, including differences in phenomenology and treatment response.

3.5 Neuroimmunology

Early reports of an association between OCD and Sydenham's chorea were confirmed in a systematic investigation (Swedo et al 1989), leading to a consideration of whether some cases of OCD involved auto-immune processes that disrupted CSTC circuits. Indeed, the term 'paediatric auto-immune neuropsychiatric disorder associated with streptococcal infections' (PANDAS) has been coined to describe patients who have acute onset of OCD symptoms and/or tics in the aftermath of streptococcal infection (Swedo et al 1998).

Table 3.2 Population and family-based genetic association studies of serotonergic candidate genes in OCD (Hemmings and Stein, 2006)

Gene (Variant)	Population	Study design	Phenotype investigated	Sample number			Result (p-values, and implicated risk allele)	References
				affected		control		
				unrelated	families			
5-HTT								
	European-American	FB	OCD		35		p < 0.03 (L^a-allele)	42
	Caucasian American	CC	OCD	75		397	p = 0.023 (LL-genotype)	43
	Jewish (Ashkenazi [A] and non-A)	CC	OCD	75 (39A)		172 (112A)	NS	44
5-HTTLPR	SA Afrikaner	CC	OCD	54		82	NS	50
	Mexican	CC/FB	OCD	115	43	136	NS	45
	Italian	CC	OCD	180		112	NS	46
	German	FB	OCD		63		NS	47
	Brazilian	CC	OCD	79		202	NS	48
	French/German	CC/FB	OCD	106	86	171	NS	49

Table 3.2 (Contd.)

Gene (Variant)	Population	Study design	Phenotype investigated	Sample number affected	Sample number control	Result (p-values, and implicated risk allele)	References
5-HT_{2A}							
−1438A/G	N. American Caucasian	CC	OCD	62	144	A-allele increased in OCD patients p < 0.05	62
	N. American Caucasian	CC	OCD	101	138	p = 0.015 and p = 0.023 (allele and genotype); A-allele in females	63
	German	CC	OCD	55	223	p = 0.046 (genotype) A-allele	64
	Mexican	CC	OCD	67	54	NS	66
	Jewish (Ashkenazi [A] and non-A)	CC	OCD	75 (39A)	172 (112A)	NS	44
T102C	Afrikaners	CC	OCD	71	129	NS	67
	SA Caucasians, stratified into Afrikaner	CC	EO[c] OCD vs. LO OCD	n(EO) = 95 [45 Afr]; n(LO) = 85 [35 Afr])		NS	68

	Population		Comparison				Ref
T102C & -1438A/G	Turkish	CC	OCD	58	83	NS	65
			OCD+tics vs. OCD-tics	n(OCD+tics) = 8		NS	
			FH (OCD) vs. no FH (OCD)	n(FH[OCD]) = 27		NS	
			SRI response vs. no SRI response	n(SRI response) = 35		NS	
C561T	Brazilian	CC	OCD	79	202	$p = 7\times10^{-5}$ (C-allele)	48
5-HT$_{2c}$							
ser23cys	Italian	CC	OCD	109	107	NS	77
			OCD+tics vs. OCD-tics	n(OCD + tics) = 23		NS	
ser23cys	Jewish (Ashkenazi [A] and non-A)	CC	OCD	75 (39A)	172 (112A)	NS	44

Table 3.2 (Contd.)

Gene (Variant)	Population	Study design	Phenotype investigated	Sample number			Result (p-values, and implicated risk allele)	Reference
				affected		control		
				unrelated	families			
5-HT_{1B}								
	Italian	FB	OCD		32		p < 0.006 (G-allele)	83
			OCD		121		p = 0.023 (G-allele)	
	Italian	FB	Age at onset (quantitative)		30		NS	84
			Y-BOCS Obsession Score		37		NS	
			Y-BOCS compulsion score		37		NS	
			Y-BOCS total score		37		NS	
G861C	Italian	FB	OCD		48		NS	85
			Y-BOCS compulsion score		48		NS	
			Y-BOCS obsession score		48		NS	
			Y-BOCS total score		48		NS	

Population	Design	Phenotype	n	Comparison	n	Significance	Ref
Afrikaners	CC	OCD	71	FH (OCD) vs. no FH (OCD)	n(FH[OCD]) = 18	NS	67
				FH (tics) vs. no FH (tics)	n(FH[tics]) = 5	NS	
				OCD+tics vs. OCD-tics	n(OCD+tics) = 9	NS	
		OCD			129	NS	
Mexican	FB	OCD	47			NS	86
		Y-BOCS compulsion score	29			NS	
		Y-BOCS obsession score	29			p = 0.034 (G-allele)	
German	FB	OCD	64			NS	47
SA Caucasians, stratified into Afrikaner (Afr)	CC	EO OCD vs. LO OCD	n(EO) = 95 [45 Afr]; n(LO) = 85 [35 Afr]			NS	68

Table 3.2 (Contd.)

Gene (Variant)	Population	Study design	Phenotype investigated	Sample number affected case unrelated	Sample number affected case families	Sample number control	Result (p-values, and implicated risk allele)	Reference
TPH								
rs1800532 (TPH1)	Jewish (Ashkenazi [A] and non-Ashkenazi)	CC	OCD	75 (39A)		172 (112A)	NS	44
	German	FB	OCD		59		NS	47
rs4570625 and rs4565946 (TPH2)	German	FB	EO OCD[d]		71		the rs4570625-rs4565946 G-C haplotype was more frequently transmitted to OCD patients (= 0.035)	89

[a] L refers to the "long" allele; [b] Studies included in meta-analysis (63) are: references 55, 56 and 63.

Abbreviations: OCD: Obsessive-compulsive disorder; **CC:** population-based case-control association; **FB:** family-based association; **NS:** non-significant finding (p>0.05); **SA:** South African; **5-HTT:** serotonin transporter; **5-HTTLPR:** variable number of tandem repeat polymorphism in the promoter region of 5-HTT, producing either long (L) or short (S) alleles.

Table 3.3 Animal Models of OCD and OCDs (adapted from Joel, 2006)

		Face validity	Predictive validity	Construct validity
		Symptom similarity	Selective Response to SRI's	Similarity of inducing mechanism/circuitry
Genetic models	D1CT-7 mice	++		+/-
	Hoxb8 mutant mice	++		+/-
	5-HT$_{2c}$ KO mice	+/-		+
	DAT KO mice	+/-		+
Pharmacological models	8-OH-DPAT-induced decrease in spontaneous alternation	+/-	++	+
	Quinpirole-induced decrease in spontaneous alternation	+/-	+	+
	Quinpirole-induced compulsive checking	+++	+	+
Behavioral models	Barbering	+++		++
	Marble burying	+	+/--	
	Signal attenuation	++	++	++

Certainly, CSTC circuits play a role in mediating the development, maintenance, and selection of procedural strategies (Saint-Cyr et al 1995; Graybiel 1998). Ventral CSTC circuits appear to play a particularly important role in recognizing behaviorally significant stimuli (and in error detection) and in regulating autonomic and goal-directed responses (including response inhibition and suppression of negative emotion) (Zald & Kim 1996; Davidson et al 2001; Rauch & Baxter 1998), and may therefore be particularly important in OCD.

It has been suggested that OCD involves a failure to inhibit CSTC-mediated procedural strategies from intruding into consciousness (Stein 2002). Such a view appears consistent with: (1) the limited number of symptom themes in OCD, and their apparent evolutionary importance; (2) dysfunction of CSTC circuits in OCD, with activation of temporal rather than striatal areas during implicit cognition (Rauch et al 2001); (3) the role of the 5-HT in particular and interrelated neurotransmitter systems in general, as the 5-HT system in CSTC circuits is thought to play an important role in mediating inhibitory processes; and (4) evidence of disinhibitory processes in OCD and related conditions (Chamberlain et al 2005).

References

Abelson, J.F., Kwan, K.Y., O'Roak, B.J., et al. (2005). Sequence variants in SLITRK1 are associated with Tourette's syndrome. *Science*, **310**: 317–320.

Adams, K.H., Hansen, E.S., Pinborg, L.H., et al. (2005). Patients with obsessive-compulsive disorder have increased 5-HT2A receptor binding in the caudate nuclei. *Int. J. Neuropsychopharmacol., J.*, **8**: 391–401.

Arnold, P.D., Rosenberg, D.R., Mundo, E., et al. (2004). Association of a glutamate (NMDA) subunit receptor gene (GRIN2B) with obsessive-compulsive disorder: a preliminary study. *Psychopharmacologia*, **174**: 530–538.

Arnold, P.D., Sicard, T., Burroughs, E., et al. (2006). Glutamate transporter gene SLC1A1 associated with obsessive-compulsive disorder. *Archs Gen. Psychiat.*, **63**: 769–776.

Azzam, A., Mathews, C.A. (2003). Meta-analysis of the association between the catecholamine-O-methyl-transferase gene and obsessive-compulsive disorder. *Am. J. Med. Genet. B Neuropsychiat. Genet.*, **123**: 64–69.

Barnes, T. D., Kubota, Y., Hu, D., et al. (2005). Activity of striatal neurons reflects dynamic encoding and recoding of procedural memories. *Nature*, **437**: 1158–1161.

Baumgarten, H.G. Grozdanovic, Z. (1998). Role of serotonin in obsessive-compulsive disorder. *Br. J. Psychiat.*, Suppl. **35**, 13–20.

Baxter, L.R., Schwartz, J.M., Bergman, K.S., et al. (1992). Caudate glucose metabolic rate changes with both drug and behavior therapy for OCD. Archs Gen. Psychiat., **49**: 681–689.

Bergqvist, P.B., Dong, J., Blier, P. (1999). Effect of atypical antipsychotic drugs on 5-HT2 receptors in the rat orbito-frontal cortex: an in vivo electrophysiological study. Psychopharmacology, **143**: 89–96.

Berridge, K.C., Aldridge, J.W., Houchard, K.R., (2005). Sequential super-stereotypy of an instinctive fixed action pattern in hyper-dopaminergic mutant mice: a model of obsessive compulsive disorder and Tourette's. BMC Biol., **3**: 4.

Brody, A.L., Saxena, S., Schwartz, J.M., FDG-PET predictors of response to behavioral therapy and pharmacotherapy in obsessive compulsive disorder. Psychiat. Res., **84**: 1–6.

Carlsson, M.L. (2001). On the role of prefrontal cortex glutamate for the antithetical phenomenology of obsessive compulsive disorder and attention deficit hyperactivity disorder. Prog. Neuropsychopharmacol. Biol. Psychiat., **25**: 5–26.

Chamberlain, S.R., Blackwell, A.D., Fineberg, N.A., et al. (2005). The neuropsychology of obsessive compulsive disorder: the importance of failures in cognitive and behavioural inhibition as candidate endophenotypic markers. Neurosci. Biobehav. Rev., **29**: 399–419.

Cheyette, S.R., Cummings, J.L. (1995). Encephalitis lethargica: lessons for contemporary neuropsychiatry. J. Neuropsychiat. Clin. Neurosci. **7**: 125–135.

Davidson, R.J., Putnam, K.M., Larson, C.L. (2001). Dysfunction in the neural circuitry of emotion regulation – a possible prelude to violence. Science, **289**: 591–594.

Delgado, P.L. Moreno, F.A. (1998). Hallucinogens, serotonin and obsessive-compulsive disorder. J. Psychoactive Drugs, **30**: 359–366.

Denys, D., van der Wee, N., Janssen, J., et al. (2004a). Low level of dopaminergic D2 receptor binding in obsessive-compulsive disorder. Biol. Psychiat., **55**: 1041–1045.

Denys, D., Zohar, J., Westenberg, H.G.M. (2004b). The role of dopamine in obsessive-compulsive disorder: preclinical and clinical evidence. J. Clin. Psychiat., **65**: 11–17.

DeVeaugh-Geiss, J., Katz, R., Landau, P. et al. (1991). Clomipramine in the treatment of patients with obsessive-compulsive disorder: the clomipramine collaborative study group. Archs Gen. Psychiat., **48**: 730–738.

Dodman, N.H., Moon-Fanelli, A., Mertens, P.A., et al. (1997) Animal models of obsessive-compulsive disorder. In Hollander, E., Stein, D.J. eds, Obsessive-Compulsive Disorders: Diagnosis, Etiology, Treatment. Marcel Dekker, New York.

Eisen, J.L., Leonard, H.L., Swedo, S.E., et al. (2001). The use of antibody D8/17 to identify B cells in adults with obsessive-compulsive disorder. Psychiat. Res., **104**: 221–225.

El Mansari, M., Bouchard, C., Blier, P. (1995). Alteration of serotonin release in the guinea pig orbito-frontal cortex by selective serotonin reuptake inhibitors. *Neuropsychopharmacology*, **13**: 117–127.

Fernandez-Cordoba, E., Lopez-Ibor Alino, J. (1967). La monoclorimi-pramina en enfermos psiquiatricos resistentes a otros tratamientos. *Acta Luso-Esp. Neurol. Psiquiat. Ciene Afines*, **26**: 119–147.

Fineberg, N.A., Gale, T.M. (2005). Evidence-based pharmacotherapy of obsessive-compulsive disorder. *Int. J. Neuropsychopharmacol.*, **8**: 107–129.

Garner, J.P., Meehan, C.L., Mench, J.A. (2003). Stereotypies in caged parrots, schizophrenia and autism: evidence for a common mechanism. *Behav. Brain Res.*, **145**: 125–134.

Garner, J.P., Weisker, S.M., Dufour, B., (2004). Barbering (fur and whisker trimming) by laboratory mice as a model of human trichotillomania and obsessive-compulsive spectrum disorders. *Comp. Med.*, **54**: 216–224.

Giedd, J.N., Rapoport, J.L., Garvey, M.A. (2000). MRI assessment of children with obsessive-compulsive disorder or tics associated with streptococcal infection. *Am. J. Psychiat.*, **157**: 281–283.

Goodman, W.K., McDougle, C.J., Lawrence, L.P. (1990). Beyond the serotonin hypothesis: a role for dopamine in some forms of obsessive-compulsive disorder. *J. Clin. Psychiat.*, **51S**: 36–43.

Gothelf, D., Presburger, G., Zohar, A.H., *et al.* (2004). Obsessive-compulsive disorder in patients with velocardiofacial (22q11 deletion) syndrome. *Am. J. Med. Genet.*, **B126**: 99–105.

Graybiel, A.M. (1998). The basal ganglia and chunking of action repertoires. *Neurobiol. Learn. Mem.*, **70**: 119–136.

Graybiel, A.M. Rauch, S.L. (2000). Toward a neurobiology of obsessive-compulsive disorder. *Neuron.*, **28**: 343–347.

Harel, Z., Hallett, J., Riggs, S., *et al.* (2001). Antibodies against human putamen in adolescents with anorexia nervosa. *Int. J. Eat. Disord.*, **29**: 463–469.

Harvey, B., Brand, A., Seedat, S., Stein, D.J. (2001). Molecular action of inositol in obsessive-compulsive disorder. *Prog. Neuropsychopharmacol. Biol. Psychiat.*

Hasler, G., Kazuba, D., Murphy, D.L. (2006). Factor analysis of obsessive-compulsive disorder YBOCS-SC symptoms and association with 5-HTTLPR SERT polymorphism. *Am. J. Med. Genet.*, **B141**: 403–408.

Hemmings, S.M.J. Stein, D.J. (2006). The current status of association studies in obsessive-compulsive disorder. *Psychiat. Clin. North Amer.*, **29**: 411–444.

Hemmings, S.M.J., Kinnear, C.J., Niehaus, D.J.H., *et al.* (2002). Dopaminergic and serotonergic system genes in obsessive-compulsive disorder: a case-control association study in the Afrikaner population. Unpublished.

Hemmings, S.M., Kinnear, C.J., Lochner, C., *et al.* (2004). Early- versus late-onset obsessive-compulsive disorder: investigating genetic and clinical correlates. *Psychiat. Res.*, **128**: 175–182.

Hettema, J.M., Neale, M.C., Kendler, K.S. (2001). A review and meta-analysis of the genetic epidemiology of anxiety disorders. *Am. J. Psychiat.*, **158**: 1568–1578.

Hugo, F., van Heerden, B., Zungu-Dirwayi, N., Stein, D.J. (1999). Functional brain imaging in obsessive-compulsive disorder secondary to neurological lesions. *Depress. Anxiety*, **10**: 129–136.

Hugo, C., Seier, J., Mdhluli, C., et al. (2003). Fluoxetine decreases stereotypic behavior in primates. *Prog. Neuropsychopharmacol. Biol. Psychiat.*, **27**: 639–643.

Ipser, J.C., Carey, P., Dhansay, Y., et al. (2006). Pharmacotherapy augmentation strategies in treatment-resistant anxiety disorders. *Cochrane Database Syst. Rev.*, CD005473.

Jenike, M.A. (1998). Neurosurgical treatment of obsessive-compulsive disorder. *Br. J. Psychiat.* Suppl. **35**: 79–90.

Joel, D. (2006). Current animal models of obsessive-compulsive disorder: a critical review. *Prog. Neuropsychopharmacol. Biol. Psychiat.*, **30**: 374–388.

Koran, L.M., Pallanti, S., Quercioli, L. (2001). Sumatriptan, 5-HT(1D) receptors and obsessive-compulsive disorder. *Eur. Neuropsychopharmacol.*, **11**: 169–172.

Leckman, J.F., Mayes, L.C. Preoccupations and behaviors associated with romantic and parental love. Perspectives on the origin of obsessive-compulsive disorder. *Child Adolesc. Psychiat. Clin. North Amer.*, **8**: 635–665.

Leonard, H.L., Swedo, S.E. (2001). Paediatric autoimmune neuropsychiatric disorders associated with streptococcal infection (PANDAS). *Int. J. Neuropsychopharmacol.* **4**: 191–198.

Lochner, C., Stein, D.J. (2001). Gender in obsessive-compulsive disorder and obsessive-compulsive spectrum disorders. *Archs Women's Mental Hlth* **4**: 19–26.

Lougee, L., Perlmutter, S.J., Nicolson, R., et al. (2000). Psychiatric disorders in first-degree relatives of children with pediatric autoimmune neuropsychiatric disorders associated with streptococcal infections (PANDAS). *J. Am. Acad. Child Adolesc. Psychiat.*, **39**: 1120–1126.

Marazziti, D., Masala, I., Rossi, A., et al. (2000). Increased inhibitory activity of protein kinase C on the serotonin transporter in OCD. *Neuropsychobiology*, **41**: 171–177.

Martin, L.J., Spicer, D.M., Lewis, M.H., et al. (1991). Social deprivation of infant monkeys alters the chemoarchitecture of the brain: I. Subcortical regions. *J. Neurosci.*, **11**: 3344–3358.

McDougle, C.J., Barr, L.C., Goodman, W.K., Price, L.H. (1999). Possible role of neuropeptides in obsessive compulsive disorder. *Psychoneuroendocrinology*, **24**: 1–24.

Merlo, L.J., Storch, E.A., Murphy, T.K., et al. (2005). Assessment of pediatric obsessive-compulsive disorder: a critical review of current methodology. *Child Psychiat. Hum. Dev.*, **36**: 195–214.

Moriarty, J., Eapen, V., Costa, D.C., et al. (1997). HMPAO SPET does not distinguish obsessive-compulsive and tic syndromes in families multiply affected with Gilles de la Tourette's syndrome. *Psychol. Med.*, **27**: 737–740.

Mundo, E., Richter, M.A., Sam, F., *et al.* (2000). Is the 5-HT(1Dbeta) receptor gene implicated in the pathogenesis of obsessive-compulsive disorder? *Am. J. Psychiat.*, **157**: 1160–1161.

Nicolini, H., Cruz, C., Paez, F., Camarena, B. (1998). Dopamine D2 and D4 receptor genes distinguish the clinical presence of tics in obsessive-compulsive disorder. *Gac. Med. Mex.*, **134**: 521–527.

Ozaki, N., Goldman, D., Kaye, W.H., *et al.* (2003). Serotonin transporter missense mutation associated with a complex neuropsychiatric phenotype. *Mol. Psychiat.*, **8**: 895, 933–895, 936.

Pato, M.T., Schindler, K.M., Pato, C.N. (2001). The genetics of obsessive-compulsive disorder. *Curr. Psychiat. Rep.*, **3**: 163–168.

Pauls, D.L., Alsobrook, J.P. 2nd. (1999). The inheritance of obsessive-compulsive disorder. *Child Adolesc. Psychiatr. Clin. North Amer.* **8**: 481–496.

Perez, J., Tardito, D., Ravizza, L., *et al.* (2000). Altered cAMP-dependent protein kinase A in platelets of patients with obsessive-compulsive disorder. *Am. J. Psychiat.*, **157**: 284–286.

Purcell, R., Maruff, P., Kyrios, M., Pantelis, C. (1998a). Cognitive deficits in obsessive-compulsive disorder on tests of frontal-striatal function. *Biol. Psychiat.*, **43**: 348–357.

Purcell, R., Maruff, P., Kyrios, M., Pantelis, C. (1998b). Neuropsychological deficits in obsessive-compulsive disorder: a comparison with unipolar depression, panic disorder, and normal controls. *Archs Gen. Psychiat.*, **55**: 415–423.

Rapoport, J.L., Ryland, D.H., Kriete, M. (1992). Drug treatment of canine acral lick. *Archs Gen. Psychiat.*, **48**: 517–521.

Rauch, S.L., Baxter, L.R.J. (1998). Neuroimaging in obsessive-compulsive disorder and related disorders. In Jenicke, M.A., Baer, L., Minichiello, W.E. eds, *Obsessive-Compulsive Disorders: Practical Management*, 3rd edn. Mosby, St Louis.

Rauch, S.L., Kim, H., Makris, N., *et al.* (2000). Volume reduction in the caudate nucleus following stereotactic placement of lesions in the anterior cingulate cortex in humans: a morphometric magnetic resonance imaging study. *J. Neurosurg.*, **2000**: 1019–1025.

Rauch, S.L., Whalen, P.J., Curran, T., *et al.* (2001). Probing striato-thalamic function in obsessive-compulsive disorder and Tourette syndrome using neuroimaging methods. *Adv. Neurol.* **85**: 207–224.

Rauch, S.L., Dougherty, D.D., Cosgrove, G.R., *et al.* (2004). What is the role of psychiatric neurosurgery in the 21st Century? *Revista Brasileira De Psiquiatria (Sao Paulo, Brazil: 1999)*, **26**: 4–5.

Ridley, R.M. (1994). The psychology of perseverative and stereotyped behavior. *Prog. Neurobiol.*, **44**: 221–231.

Rosenberg, D.R., Keshavan, M.S. (1998). Toward a neurodevelopmental model of obsessive-compulsive disorder. *Biol. Psychiat.*, **43**: 623–640.

Rosenberg, D.R., MacMillan, S.N., Moore, G.J. (2001). Brain anatomy and chemistry may predict treatment response in paediatric obsessive-compulsive disorder. *Int. J. Neuropsychopharmacol.*, **4**: 179–190.

Saint-Cyr, J.A., Taylor, A.E., Nicholson, K. (1995). Behavior and the basal ganglia. Weiner, W.J., Lang, A.E. eds, *Behavioral Neurology of Movement Disorders*. Raven Press, New York.

Saxena, S., Brody, A.L., Maidment, K.M., et al. (2004). Cerebral glucose metabolism in obsessive-compulsive hoarding. *Am. J. Psychiat.*, **161**: 1038–1048.

Shapira, N.A., Liu, Y., He, A.G., et al. (2003). Brain activation by disgust-inducing pictures in obsessive-compulsive disorder. *Biol. Psychiat.*, **54**: 751–756.

Shugart, Y.Y., Samuels, J., Willour, V.L., et al. (2006). Genomewide linkage scan for obsessive-compulsive disorder: evidence for susceptibility loci on chromosomes 3q, 7p, 1q, 15q, and 6q. *Mol. Psychiat.*, **11**: 763–770.

Simpson, H.B., Lombardo, I., Slifstein, M., et al. (2003). Serotonin transporters in obsessive-compulsive disorder: a positron emission tomography study with [(11)C]McN 5652. *Biol. Psychiat.*, **54**: 1414–1421.

Snider, L.A., Lougee, L., Slattery, M., et al. (2005). Antibiotic prophylaxis with azithromycin or penicillin for childhood-onset neuropsychiatric disorders. *Biol. Psychiat.*, **57**: 788–792.

Stein, D.J. (1999). Single photon emission computed tomography of the brain with tc-99m HMPAO during sumatriptan challenge in obsessive-compulsive disorder: investigating the functional role of the serotonin auto-receptor. *Prog. Neuropsychopharmacol. Biol. Psychiat.*, **23**: 1079–1099.

Stein, D.J. (2002). Seminar on obsessive-compulsive disorder. *Lancet*, **360**: 397–405.

Stein, D.J., Hollander, E., Cohen, L. (1994). Neuropsychiatry of obsessive-compulsive disorder. In Hollander, E., Zohar, J., Marazziti, D., and Olivier, B. eds, *Current Insights in Obsessive-Compulsive Disorder*. Wiley, Chichester.

Stein, D.J., Goodman, W.K., Rauch, S.L. (2000). The cognitive-affective neuroscience of obsessive-compulsive disorder. *Curr. Psychiat. Rep.*, **2**: 341–346.

Stein, D.J., Liu, Y., Shapira, N.A., Goodman, W. K. (2001). The psychobiology of obsessive-compulsive disorder: how important is the role of disgust? *Curr. Psychiat. Rep.* **3**: 281–287.

Stern, L., Zohar, J., Cohen, R., Sasson, Y. (1998). Treatment of severe, drug resistant obsessive compulsive disorder with the 5HT1D agonist sumatriptan. *Eur. Neuropsychopharmacol.*, **8**: 325–328.

Swedo, S.E., Leonard, H.L., Garvey, M., et al. (1998). Pediatric autoimmune neuropsychiatric disorders associated with streptococcal infections: clinical description of the first 50 cases. *Am. J. Psychiat.*, **155**: 264–271.

Swedo, S.E., Rapoport, J.L., Cheslow, D.L., et al. (1989). High prevalence of obsessive-compulsive symptoms in patients with Sydenham's chorea. *Am. J. Psychiat.*, **146**: 246–249.

Swedo, S.E., Grant, P.J. (2005). Annotation: PANDAS: a model for human autoimmune disease. *J. Child Psychol. Psychiat. Allied Discipl.*, **46**: 227–234.

Szeszko, P.R., Robinson, D., Alvir, J.M.J., *et al.* (1999). Orbital frontal and amygdala volume reductions in obsessive-compulsive disorder. *Archs. Gen. Psychiat.*, **56**: 913–919.

Talbot, P.S. (2004). The molecular neuroimaging of anxiety disorders. *Curr. Psychiat. Rep.*, **6**, 274–279.

Thoren, P., Asberg, M., Bertilsson, L. (1980). Clomipramine treatment of obsessive-compulsive disorder. II. Biochemical aspects. *Archs Gen. Psychiat.*, **37**: 1289–1294.

Urraca, N., Camarena, B., Gomez-Caudillo, L., *et al.* (2004). Mu opioid receptor gene as a candidate for the study of obsessive-compulsive disorder with and without tics. *Am. J. Med. Genet.*, **B127**: 94–96.

van der Wee, N. J., Stevens, H., Hardeman, J.A., *et al.* (2004). Enhanced dopamine transporter density in psychotropic-naive patients with obsessive-compulsive disorder shown by [123I] beta -CIT SPECT. *Am. J. Psychiat.*, **161**: 2201–2206.

van Grootheest, D.S., Cath, D.C., Beekman, A.T., Boomsma, D.I. (2005). Twin studies on obsessive-compulsive disorder: a review. *Twin Res. Hum. Genet.*, **8**: 450–458.

Whiteside, S.P., Port, J.D., Abramowitz, J.S. (2004). A meta-analysis of functional neuroimaging in obsessive-compulsive disorder. *Psychiat. Res.*, **132**: 69–79.

Williams, K.E., Koran, L.M. (1997). Obsessive-compulsive disorder in pregnancy, the puerperium, and the premenstruum. *J. Clin. Psychiat.*, **58**: 330–334.

Zai, G., Arnold, P., Burroughs, E., *et al.* (2005). Evidence for the gamma-amino-butyric acid type B receptor 1 (GABBR1) gene as a susceptibility factor in obsessive-compulsive disorder. *Am. J. Med. Genet.*, **134**: 25–29.

Zai, G., Bezchlibnyk, Y.B., Richter, M.A., *et al.* (2004). Myelin oligodendro-cyte glycoprotein (MOG) gene is associated with obsessive-compulsive disorder. *Am. J. Med. Genet.*, **B129**: 64–68.

Zald, D.H., Kim, S.W. (1996). Anatomy and function of the orbital frontal cortex, I: Anatomy, neurocircuitry, and obsessive-compulsive disorder. *J. Neuropsychiat. Clin. Neurosci.*, **8**: 125–138.

Zohar, J., Insel, T.R., Zohar-Kadouch, R.C. (1988). Serotonergic responsiv-ity in obsessive-compulsive disorder: Effects of chronic clomipramine treatment. *Archs Gen. Psychiat.*, **45**: 167–172.

Zohar, J., Insel, T.R. (1987). Drug treatment of obsessive-compulsive disorder. *J. Affect. Disord.*, **13**: 193–202.

Zuchner, S., Cuccaro, M.L., Tran-Viet, K.N., *et al.* (2006). SLITRK1 muta-tions in Trichotillomania. *Mol. Psychiat.*, **11**: 888–889.

Zungu-Dirwayi, N., Hugo, F., van Heerden, B.B., Stein, D.J. (1999). Are musical obsessions a temporal lobe phenomenon? *J. Neuropsychiat. Clin. Neurosci.*, **11**: 398–400.

Chapter 4

Pharmacotherapy

> ### Key points
> - First-line treatment should be with selective serotonin reuptake inhibitors (SSRIs) for most cases
> - The treatment effect emerges slowly and gradually over weeks and months
> - Long-term treatment protects against relapse
> - Strategies for SRI-resistant obsessive-compulsive disorder (OCD) are under investigation

4.1 The pharmacological specificity of OCD

The weight of evidence shows that OCD responds preferentially to drugs which powerfully inhibit the synaptic reuptake of serotonin (serotonin reuptake inhibitors; SRIs). These are the:

- Tricyclic antidepressant clomipramine.
- More highly selective serotonin reuptake inhibitors (SSRIs).

Randomized controlled trials have shown that these drugs are clinically effective treatments for OCD, both in the presence and absence of comorbid depression (reviewed in Fineberg & Gale 2005). In contrast, despite occasional positive trials, other classes of medication (monoamine oxidase inhibitors, benzodiazepines, dopamine blockers) have not consistently been found effective (Box 4.1). This selective pharmacological response has generated hypotheses about the role of serotonin in the aetiology of OCD but, so far, no unifying theory has been proved (see Chapter 3), and the mechanisms by which SSRIs exert anti-obsessional benefits remain only partially understood (Fineberg et al 1997).

> ## Box 4.1 The pharmacological specificity of obsessive-compulsive disorder (Fineberg & Gale 2005)
>
> *Effective*
> - Potent SRIs e.g.
>   - clomipramine
>   - fluvoxamine
>   - fluoxetine
>   - sertraline
>   - paroxetine
>   - citalopram
>   - escitalopram
>
> *Ineffective*
> - Tricyclics (apart from clomipramine)
> - Monoamine oxidase inhibitors
> - Lithium
> - Benzodiazepines
> - Buspirone
> - Electroconvulsive therapy
>
> *Potentially effective in combination with SRIs:*
> - Conventional antipsychotics e.g. haloperidol
> - Atypical antipsychotics e.g. olanzapine, quetiapine, risperidone
> - Clonazepam

4.2 Clomipramine

Building on several small, positive trials (reviewed in Fineberg & Gale 2005), two seminal multicentre studies of clomipramine for non-depressed adult patients with OCD (de Veaugh-Geiss *et al* 1989, Clomipramine Collaborative Study Group 1991) and one for childhood OCD (De Veaugh-Geiss *et al* 1992) were performed early on. Significant differences between drug and placebo emerged in favour of clomipramine as early as the first week of treatment. However, the benefits of clomipramine, given in flexible doses, continued to increase slowly and gradually over several weeks.

4.3 Selective serotonin reuptake inhibitors

The introduction of SSRIs provided the potential for agents that were not only effective for OCD but that also had a superior safety and tolerability profile to clomipramine. The efficacy of fluvoxamine, sertraline, fluoxetine, paroxetine, citalopram and escitalopram in the treatment of OCD has been demonstrated unequivocally in large-scale acute-phase studies (described in detail below). Several SSRIs have also been shown effective in paediatric OCD, some from the age of 7 years onwards. Like clomipramine, the treatment effect increases gradually over many weeks. Although clomipramine is a powerful SRI, it has an active metabolite with strong noradrenergic properties. That the more highly selective SSRIs are also beneficial, showing a similar, incremental effect, suggests that their anti-obsessional actions are related to their SRI properties.

4.3.1 **Placebo-controlled trials of fluvoxamine**
4.3.1.1 *Adults*

Small double-blind studies, some employing a crossover design (Perse et al 1987), demonstrated similar efficacy in depressed and non-depressed OCD patients (Goodman et al 1989; Jenike et al 1990a). In the study by Cottraux et al (1990) fluvoxamine also showed superiority over placebo in spite of concurrent exposure therapy in the placebo group. The multicentre placebo-controlled study by Goodman et al (1996) confirmed superiority for fluvoxamine (100–300mg). Obsessions and compulsions both improved, with a possible earlier benefit for obsessions. Another multicentre study demonstrated efficacy for controlled-release (CR) fluvoxamine (100–300mg; Hollander et al 2003a).

4.3.1.2 *Children*

Riddle et al (2001) demonstrated efficacy for fluvoxamine (50–200mg) in 120 children aged 8–17 years. Only three patients on fluvoxamine and one on placebo withdrew through adverse effects. This finding suggests efficacy and tolerability for fluvoxamine in childhood OCD.

4.3.2 **Placebo-controlled trials of sertraline**
4.3.2.1 *Adults*

Placebo-controlled studies by Chouinard et al (1990), Kronig et al (1999) and a multicentre trial by Greist et al (1995a) demonstrated efficacy for sertraline in daily doses ranging from 50 to 200mg. Jenike et al (1990b) found no group differences in a study that was arguably underpowered.

4.3.2.2 *Children*

March et al (1998) found a significant advantage over placebo for sertraline, titrated up to 200mg, in a cohort of children and adolescents. Cardiovascular parameters showed no clinically meaningful abnormalities. Although insomnia, nausea, agitation and tremor occurred more often in the drug-treated group, only 13% of sertraline patients discontinued early because of adverse effects (cf. 3% placebo), suggesting that sertraline is safe up to doses of 200mg in children (Wilens et al 1999). In the Pediatric OCD Treatment Study (POTS, 2004) children and adolescents received cognitive-behavioural therapy (CBT) alone, sertraline alone, combined CBT and sertraline, or pill placebo. All three active treatments appeared acceptable and well-tolerated, with no evidence of treatment-emergent harm to self or to others. The lack of a matched control treatment for CBT limited conclusions about relative efficacy: sertraline alone, and in combination with CBT, was efficacious compared with pill placebo.

A pooled analysis of the childhood OCD studies comparing 'numbers needed to treat' with those 'needed to harm' revealed no suicidal actions and a positive risk ratio for the use of sertraline in children and adolescents with OCD (March et al 2006).

4.3.3 **Placebo-controlled trials of fluoxetine**

4.3.3.1 *Adults*

Two multicentre studies benefited from a design that allowed comparison of different fixed doses. In the study by Montgomery et al (1993), the 20mg dose fared no better than placebo, while the 40mg dose and the 60mg dose were superior. In the larger, longer study by Tollefson et al (1994), all fixed doses of fluoxetine emerged as superior to placebo but there was a trend toward superiority for the 60mg dose. In a placebo-controlled active comparator study (Jenike et al 1997), fluoxetine was superior to placebo and also to the mono-amine oxidase inhibitor phenelzine, which did not differentiate from placebo.

4.3.3.2 *Children*

Three studies have looked at fluoxetine in childhood OCD, all showing superiority over placebo. Riddle et al's (1992) crossover study used fixed doses of 20mg. Behavioural activation occurred as an adverse effect in a few children, and one left the study early because of suicidal ideation. The authors considered these side-effects to be dose-related and advocated initiating treatment at doses lower than 20mg/day. Geller et al (2001) took a larger cohort, titrating doses upwards from 10 to 60mg over 13 weeks. Fluoxetine was superior to placebo and well-tolerated, with similar dropout rates from adverse events on drug and placebo. In the trial by Leibowitz et al (2002) the dose-range was extended to 80mg after the first 6 weeks. After 8 weeks, responders could continue double-blind treatment for a further 8 weeks. No patient withdrew from adverse effects. These results suggest fluoxetine is clinically effective across the dose range in children with OCD.

4.3.4 **Placebo-controlled trials of paroxetine**

4.3.4.1 *Adults*

The multicentre study by Zohar and Judge (1996) included clomipramine as a comparator agent. Paroxetine, given in doses up to 60mg, was significantly more effective than placebo and of comparable efficacy to clomipramine (50–250mg). In another large trial, Hollander et al (2003b) tested paroxetine in fixed doses (20mg,

40mg and 60mg) with placebo. Both higher doses significantly outper-formed both placebo and the 20mg dose which did not separate from placebo. The comparator study by Stein et al (2007), which was extended up to 24 weeks, included a 40mg fixed-dose arm which showed efficacy against placebo at the 12 and 24-week rating points.

4.3.4.2 Children

Geller et al (2004) reported efficacy for paroxetine (10–50mg) in a study of 204 children and adolescents from as young as 7 years. Paroxetine was generally well tolerated: 10.2% of patients in the paro-xetine group and 2.9% in the placebo group discontinued treatment because of adverse events.

4.3.5 Placebo-controlled trials of citalopram

4.3.5.1 Adults

The multinational placebo-controlled study by Montgomery et al (2001) showed efficacy for fixed doses of 20mg, 40mg and 60mg citalopram compared with placebo. Citalopram was well tolerated and improved psychosocial disability on the Sheehan Disability Scale (Sheehan et al 1996).

4.3.6 Placebo-controlled studies of escitalopram

4.3.6.1 Adults

Escitalopram, an SSRI with dual actions on the serotonin transporter (Sanchez et al 2004), was investigated in a multicentre, active-referenced study which extended for as long as 24 weeks (Stein et al 2007). Patients were randomized to escitalopram 10mg/day, escitalo-pram 20mg/day, paroxetine 40mg/day or placebo. After 12 weeks, both 20mg escitalopram and paroxetine were superior to placebo, and by week 24 all three active treatments were superior. These results highlight the importance of continuing treatment beyond the acute phase. They suggest escitalopram (10–20mg) is effective, with a faster onset of action for the 20mg dose.

4.3.7 Which SRI is most clinically effective?

Clinical effectiveness usually depends upon a balance between efficacy, safety and tolerability.

Practice point: When deciding upon a drug treatment ...
Consider efficacy, safety and tolerability.

So far, only three controlled studies have compared the clinical effectiveness of different SSRIs, and the results were not strong enough to support the superior efficacy of any one compound (Mundo et al 1997a; Bergeron et al 2001; Stein et al 2007).

SSRIs are generally safe and well-tolerated, according to the placebo-referenced treatment trials which reported adverse-event-related withdrawal rates of around 5–15%. As a group, SSRIs cause unwanted nausea, insomnia, somnolence, dizziness and diarrhoea. Sexual side-effects include reduced libido and delayed orgasm, and can also affect up to 30% of individuals (Monteiro et al 1987).

When choosing a particular SSRI the clinician should take account of pharmacokinetic variation which may result in unwanted interactions with other drugs being prescribed. In this respect, fluoxetine, paroxetine and to a much lesser extent sertraline, inhibit the P450 isoenzyme CYP 2D6 which metabolizes tricyclic antidepressants, antipsychotics, anti-arrythmics and beta-blockers, whereas fluvoxamine inhibits both CYP 1A2 and CYP 3A4, which eliminate warfarin, tricyclics, benzodiazepines and some anti-arrhythmics. Citalopram and escitalopram are relatively free from hepatic interactions. Fluoxetine has a long half-life, and fewer discontinuation effects, which can be advantageous for patients who forget to take their tablets. It has also been extensively used in pregnancy and generally shown to be safe (Bairy et al 2007).

Head-to-head studies have demonstrated that whereas the SRIs appear equally efficacious in treating OCD, SSRIs are tolerated better than clomipramine (Table 4.1). For example, in the study of Zohar & Judge (1996), the dropout rate from adverse effects on clomipramine (17%) was higher than for paroxetine (9%). Rouillon et al (1998) also reported that clomipramine was associated with significantly more withdrawals associated with side-effects than fluvoxamine, and in the analysis by Bisserbe et al (1997) superior tolerability of sertraline over clomipramine produced a greater over-all benefit.

Clomipramine can also be associated with potentially dangerous side-effects. Cardiotoxicity and cognitive impairment occur substantially more with clomipramine than with SSRIs. In addition there is an increased risk of convulsions in patients taking clomipramine (up to 2%). Overdose on clomipramine can prove fatal, and this needs to be borne in mind when prescribing for OCD, in view of the elevated suicide risk associated with the illness. Clomipramine is also associated with greater impairment of sexual performance (up to 80% of patients) compared with SSRIs (up to 30% of patients; Monteiro et al 1987), weight gain (Maina et al 2003a) and troublesome anticholinergic effects. On the other hand, SSRIs are associated with initially increased nausea, nervousness, and insomnia.

Table 4.1 Controlled studies comparing SSRIs with clomipramine (CMI)

Drug and study	n	Design	Outcome Efficacy	Tolerability
Fluoxetine (FLX)				
Pigott et al (1990)	11	CMI (50–250mg) vs FLX (20–80mg)	CMI = FLX	FLX > CMI
Lopez-Ibor et al (1996)	30 vs 24	CMI 150mg vs FLX 40mg	CMI = FLX on primary criterion / CMI > FLX on other criteria	FLX = CMI
Fluvoxamine (FLV)				
Smeraldi et al (1992)	10	CMI 200mg vs FLV 220mg	CMI = FLV	FLV = CMI
Freeman et al (1994)	30 vs 34	CMI (150–250mg) vs FLV (150–250mg)	CMI = FLV	FLV > CMI (on severe effects)
Korar et al (1996)	42 vs 37	CMI (100–250mg) vs FLV (100–250mg)	CMI = FLV	FLV = CMI
Milanfranchi et al (1997)	13 vs 13	CMI (50–300mg) vs FLV (50–300mg)	CMI = FLV	FLV = CMI
Rouillon (1998)	105 vs 112	CMI (150–300mg) vs FLV (150–300mg)	CMI = FLV	FLV > CMI
Paroxetine (PAR)				
Zohar & Judge (1996)	99 vs 201 vs 99	CMI (50–250mg) vs PAR (20–60mg) vs placebo	CMI > placebo / PAR > placebo	PAR > CMI
Sertraline (SER)				
Bisserbe et al (1997)	82 vs 86	CMI (50–200mg) vs SER (50–200mg)	SER = CMI	SER > CMI

Practice points: When choosing an SRI for OCD ...

- Use an SSRI first-line for most cases.
- Check for potential drug interactions and select SSRI accordingly.
- Check for potential suicidal behaviour.
- Choose clomipramine for those who fail treatment with SSRIs or who cannot tolerate them.

4.3.8 **Meta-analyses of SRIs**

Meta-analyses combine data from separate studies using specific rules. They can provide a more objective and quantifiable measure of treatment-effect size than narrative reviews. However, they are subject to the confounding effects of imbalances in populations studied, differing severities, and differing methodology for each study, so results for analyses on the OCD trials, which spanned several decades, must be viewed with a great deal of caution (Pigott & Seay 1999). There is also the risk that a significant difference reported in a large meta-analysis may reflect only a small difference between the treatments, which may not be clinically relevant. For these reasons the evidence from meta-analyses is considered weaker than evidence from individual controlled studies. In short, meta-analyses cannot substitute for high-quality head-to-head comparator trials.

Meta-analysis of OCD trials introduced the idea that less 'serotonin selective' agents such as clomipramine might have a greater effect size than SSRIs: whereas most meta-analyses demonstrated significant advantages for all SRIs over placebo, some showed superiority for clomipramine over SSRIs which were more or less comparable (Jenike et al 1990a; Stein et al 1995; Piccinelli et al 1995; Greist et al 1995b; Abramowitz 1997; Kobak et al 1998; Ackerman & Greenland 2002). Variation between individual studies in factors such as year of publication, length of single-blind pre-randomization period, length of trial, severity of OCD, and the recent rise in placebo-response rates were acknowledged to have potentially biased the results in favour of clomipramine.

The UK National Collaborating Centre for Mental Health systematically accessed unpublished as well as published randomized studies, which were included in their meta-analysis only if they met stringent methodological criteria, as part of the UK National Institute for Health and Clinical Excellence (NICE) comprehensive treatment guideline (NICE 2006). Clomipramine and SSRIs could not be distinguished in terms of efficacy whereas there was some limited evidence suggesting that clomipramine was associated with a higher rate of adverse-events-related, premature trial discontinuations than SSRIs (www.nice.org.uk).

Geller et al (2003a) performed a meta-analysis on pharmacotherapy for childhood OCD. The results were consistent with the adult literature. In the absence of head-to-head studies, the authors recommended that clomipramine should not generally be used first-line in children because of its more problematic side-effect profile. Fineberg et al (2004) directly compared SRI treatment trials in childhood OCD with those in adult OCD in a meta analysis. Effect sizes overlapped for children and adults, to the extent that it was not possible to discriminate between the efficacy and tolerability of SRIs in children and adults with OCD. These results imply a similar treatment response for childhood and adulthood OCD.

4.3.9 **Which dose?**

Dose-finding studies have suggested that higher doses (20mg escitalopram; 60mg citalopram, fluoxetine, paroxetine; 200mg sertraline) are more effective, although the evidence for higher doses of sertraline and citalopram was less clear cut (reviewed in Fineberg et al 2005). Clomipramine and fluvoxamine have not been investigated using fixed-dose comparator groups. The study by Montgomery (1980) did show efficacy for a relatively low fixed dose of 75mg clomipramine. Table 4.2 shows recommended dose-ranges for SSRIs in OCD.

4.3.10 **Dose titration**

Fast upwards titration may produce earlier responses, but the long-term benefits of this approach are unclear. A single-blind study compared rapid dose-escalation with sertraline to 150mg over 5 days, with slower dose-escalation over 15 days, and found an early advantage for the rapid titration group which disappeared after week 6 (Bogetto et al 2002). In another study, pulse loading with intravenous clomipramine produced a large and rapid decrease in obsessive symptoms, but oral pulse loading did not, and the early advantages were not sustained over treatment (Koran et al 1997). In contrast,

Table 4.2 Recommended dose ranges of SSRIs for adult OCD*	
Medication	Dose range
Citalopram	20–60mg/day
Escitalopram	10–20mg/day
Fluoxetine	20–80mg/day
Fluvoxamine	50–300mg/day
Paroxetine	20–60mg/day
Sertraline	50–200mg/day

* For children and adolescents (aged 8–16 years) starting at half the lowest listed dose is advisable.

the escitalopram dose-finding study (Stein *et al* 2007) showed that although slower than the 20mg dose, the 10mg dose eventually did reach efficacy after 24 weeks.

The arguments for slower dose-increases are persuasive, particularly in children and the elderly. Early SSRI-related adverse effects such as nausea and agitation can be ameliorated by slowly titrating upwards over weeks and months. Particular care with higher doses is required for cases with comorbidity. For example, patients with comorbid panic disorder may be particularly sensitive to early anxiogenic effects of SSRIs and lower than average doses may be required for the first week or two. Those with bipolar affective disorder are susceptible to switching into mania and may require additional mood stabilizers. Longer-term side-effects such as sleep disturbance and headache are also dose-related, and need to be monitored. Sexual dysfunction is a common cause of drug discontinuation, and, if necessary, strategies such as dose reduction, short drug holidays or use of drugs with restorative potency (e.g. viagra, mianserin (Aizenberg *et al* 1999)) can be considered in stable cases.

4.3.11 **The response to SRI is slow and gradual**

Patients should be warned, at the outset of treatment with clomipramine or an SSRI, that the anti-obsessional effect takes several weeks to develop fully. Sometimes progress seems remarkably slow, and patients may find it difficult to acknowledge changes are occurring. It may be helpful to recruit family or friends to substantiate these improvements.

Side-effects such as nausea and agitation tend to emerge early, before signs of improvement are consolidated, but usually abate over time. However, placebo-referenced gains accrue for at least 6 months (Stein *et al* 2007) and, according to open-label follow-up data, for at least 2 years (Rasmussen *et al* 1997). It is important, therefore, to allow time for the treatment effect to develop and not to discontinue or change the drug prematurely. A trial of at least 12 weeks at the maximum tolerated dose and careful assessment is advisable before judging its effectiveness. Although response to medication does not necessarily imply symptom remission, it is usually associated with significant improvement in quality of life (Tenney *et al* 2003; Stein *et al* 2007).

4.3.12 **Response and remission on SRI treatment**

The response to treatment with SRI is characteristically partial, at least in the early stages. There is general agreement that reduction in Yale–Brown Obsessive Compulsive Scale (Y-BOCS) scores of around 25% from baseline represent a clinically relevant improvement. In placebo-controlled trials between 30 and 60% cases reached this level of clinical response within the acute treatment phase

(Fineberg & Gale 2005). However, it is important to recognize that the patients studied in randomized controlled trials are often drawn from centres specializing in OCD, which result in lower response rates because more treatment-resistant patients are seen at such sites. Open-label studies are usually associated with higher rates of SRI response than placebo trials because all patients know they are receiving active treatment.

Practice points: When starting treatment with an SRI ...

- Check for comorbidity that might impact on the initial dose.
- For most adult patients start treatment with average doses (children and adolescents start with lower doses).
- Advise the patient that the treatment effect comes on slowly, and that many side effects will abate with time.
- Recruit family member or friend to help assess treatment response.
- Increase dose gradually, at intervals of several weeks, titrating upwards against clinical response, to maximal recommended doses.
- Continue for at least 12 weeks at maximal tolerated dose level before judging effectiveness.
- Remission and recovery are potentially achievable goals.

The concept of remission for OCD is more debatable and there is no universally accepted definition. It has been described as a brief period during which sufficient improvement has occurred that the individual no longer suffers with OCD, while recovery represents a long-lasting remission (Simpson et al 2006). Studies have chosen remission criteria ranging from Y-BOCS ≤16 to Y-BOCS ≤7 and have demonstrated that remission can be achieved on SSRI in up to 50% of cases (Simpson et al 2006; Stein et al 2007).

4.3.13 **What if patients do not respond on SRIs?**

4.3.13.1 *Review diagnosis and compliance*

Failure to respond should alert the clinician to the possibility of misdiagnosis. Tourette's syndrome and Asperger's syndrome are just two OCD-related disorders that can easily be mistaken for OCD, while alcohol abuse may be hidden. Adherence to the drug-regimen should also be confirmed. It can be helpful to measure drug plasma levels. For example, rapid metabolizers of SRIs might respond less well. It is not clear how common a problem this might be in the OCD population. For patients with OCD, various negative clinical predictors have been described, including hoarding symptoms, comorbid tics, and schizotypal personality disorder – consistent with evidence that the dopamine system is important in their mediation.

Following poor response to an adequate trial of SRI, the clinician has a variety of options (Figure 4.1). The evidence supporting these approaches is not as strong as for first-line treatments and relies on small-scale trials. Switching to a different SSRI or clomipramine is the usual first step. Subsequently, one may consider adding an anti-psychotic agent, or elevating the dose of SRI (perhaps particularly relevant when there has been a partial response). Alternative options include changing the mode of delivery or introducing novel agents. The clinician should weigh up the relative advantages and disadvantages of these approaches and discuss them with the patient before proceeding.

4.3.13.2 Adding a dopamine blocker

For truly SRI-resistant cases the strongest evidence supports adding low doses of dopamine blockers to existing SRI therapy; earlier placebo-controlled randomized trials were undertaken with first generation antipsychotics, and more recent studies (reviewed in Fineberg et al 2006) including meta-analyses (Fineberg et al 2006a; Ipser et al 2006) have confirmed the effectiveness of the better-tolerated new generation antipsychotic agents such as olanzapine (around 10mg), quetiapine (200–300mg) and risperidone (2–4mg) in adults. Another meta-analysis (Bloch et al 2006) concluded that SRI-refractory patients with comorbid tics responded particularly well to adding antipsychotics.

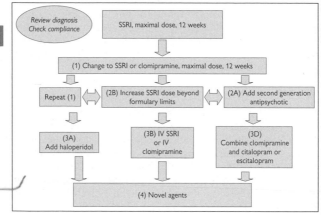

Figure 4.1 Serotonin reuptake inhibitor (SRI)-resistant obsessive-compulsive disorder: a treatment algorithm

More studies are needed to determine the relative effectiveness of different antipsychotic agents and doses. We suggest starting with low doses (around 0.5mg risperidone, 50mg quetiapine) and titrating upwards gradually, monitoring for clinical response and side-effects. Longer-term studies are also needed to clarify long-term efficacy and risks of metabolic side-effects. Second generation antipsychotics such as risperidone and quetiapine may currently be preferred as the first-line strategy, since they are generally well-tolerated in the context of short-term efficacy trials. Weight gain has been reported in trials of olanzapine (Bystritsy et al 2004) and drowsiness in trials of olanzapine (Bystritsky et al 2004) and quetiapine (Fineberg et al 2005). It remains uncertain as to how long patients should remain on augmented treatment: a small retrospective study by Maina et al (2003b) showed that the majority of patients who had responded to the addition of an antipsychotic to their SRI subsequently relapsed when the antipsychotic was withdrawn.

4.3.14 Increasing SRI dose above normal limits

4.3.14.1 SSRI
Uncontrolled case reports suggest that individuals who have tolerated maximal doses of SSRI without adverse reactions may benefit from further increasing SSRI doses above formulary limits without adverse effects developing [e.g. citalopram 160mg/day (Bejerot & Bodland 1998), sertraline 400mg/day (Byerly et al 1996)]. It is not yet possible to predict which individuals might respond best to this strategy, nor how high the dose should be. There would seem to be reasonable grounds for gradually and cautiously increasing daily doses of SSRI if the patient is in good physical health, the SSRI is well tolerated, and plasma levels turn out to be low. Patients need to be advised that the proposed dose exceeds usual recommended limits.

4.3.14.2 Clomipramine
For clomipramine, doses up to 300mg have been systematically investigated and found to be acceptable (De Veaugh Geiss et al 1989). However, given its propensity to produce anticholinergic side-effects, a high risk of convulsions (up to 2%) and potentially dangerous cardiotoxicity, doses of clomipramine exceeding this level should usually be avoided unless electrocardiogram (ECG) and plasma-level monitoring is available. Trough plasma levels of clomipramine combined with its metabolite desmethylclompiramine should usually be kept below 450ng/ml to minimize toxicity (Szegedi et al 1996).

4.3.14.3 Intravenous clomipramine
Results from a controlled study support the use of intravenous clomipramine in adults resistant to oral treatment (Fallon et al 1998), but this may not always be practical since on-hand resuscitation facilities are required.

4.3.14.4 *SRI combinations*

Combinations of SRIs have been found useful in some studies (Pallanti *et al* 1999). However, caution is required if clomipramine is to be combined with SSRIs that potentially cross-react at the hepatic microsomes, and plasma-level and ECG monitoring are usually recommended. Citalopram, escitalopram (and to a lesser extent sertraline) are unlikely to interfere with the clearance of clomipramine and are therefore preferred for this approach.

4.3.14.5 *Other compounds*

A range of augmenting agents from other classes (e.g. lithium, buspirone, pindolol, inositol) has been studied in controlled trials in adulthood OCD, but to date, findings have been negative or inconsistent. Agents with significant serotonin reuptake inhibition, such as venlafaxine, may be effective in OCD, but further work is needed to demonstrate this. Recent positive case reports for drugs acting at the N-methyl-D-asparate receptors such as riluzole (Coric *et al* 2005) and memantine (Poyurovsky *et al* 2005) merit systematic investigation under double-blind conditions.

4.4 Is long-term pharmacological treatment beneficial?

Obsessive-compulsive disorder is a chronic illness and so treatment needs to keep the patient well over the longer term. A small number of double-blind studies lasting up to 12 months have shown that those who responded to acute treatment benefited from continuing with medication with no evidence of tolerance developing. In the study by Tollefson *et al* (1994), patients on all doses of fluoxetine (20, 40, 60mg) continued to improve, but additional significant improvements were evident for the 60mg group only, suggesting added benefit for remaining at the higher dose level. In the larger extension study by Greist *et al* (1995a), patients who had responded to 12 weeks treatment with sertraline or placebo continued under double-blind conditions for 40 weeks. Improvements were sustained for those who remained on sertraline, and side-effects improved over time. Fifty-nine completers were followed up for a further year on open-label sertraline, and showed significant additional improvements in OCD symptoms over the course of the second year, with a reduced incidence of side-effects compared with the earlier study (Rasmussen *et al* 1997).

4.4.1 How long should treatment continue?

One way of tackling this question is to explore whether continuation of treatment provides ongoing benefit and protects against relapse. Studies looking at the short-term effects of discontinuing clomipramine or SSRIs under double-blind, placebo-controlled conditions showed a rapid and incremental worsening of symptoms in people who switched to placebo (reviewed in Fineberg & Gale 2005).

4.4.2 Relapse prevention trials

Relapse prevention studies are difficult to conduct, and the results of studies so far have been mixed, largely owing to methodological problems. The design involves selecting responders to open-label drug and then randomizing them either to continuation or to placebo (Table 4.3). In the fluoxetine study by Romano et al (2001), patients remaining on the highest dose (60mg) showed significantly lower relapse rates (17.5%), implying an ongoing advantage for staying at the higher dose levels, but the study still did not discriminate between continuation of pooled fluoxetine and discontinuation. In spite of its larger size and longer duration, the study by Koran et al (2002) was also unable to demonstrate a significant advantage for sertraline on the a-priori criterion for preventing relapse; in this case almost certainly because the criterion for relapse was too strictly defined. However, those remaining on sertraline showed significantly fewer "dropouts due to relapse or insufficient clinical response" and "acute exacerbation of symptoms", and ongoing sertraline was associated with continued improvement in Y-BOCS scores and quality-of-life measures. In a study of children and adolescents (Geller et al 2003b), the overall relapse rate was not significantly higher in the placebo than paroxetine group (43.9 versus 34.7%), possibly because the duration of follow-up was too short. However, the large-scale study of paroxetine by Hollander et al (2003b) clearly demonstrated a significantly better outcome for those remaining on the active drug over the 6-month double-blind discontinuation phase: 59% of patients randomized to placebo relapsed, compared to 38% remaining on paroxetine (20–60mg), with paroxetine being well-tolerated long-term. In another large relapse prevention study using escitalopram (10–20mg), patients randomized to placebo relapsed significantly earlier. After 24 weeks, 52% placebo cases had relapsed, compared with 24% on escitalopram and the risk of relapsing on placebo was 2.7 times higher compared to escitalopram (Fineberg et al 2006c).

4.4.3 Relapse prevention as a treatment target

Taken together these results suggest that relapse prevention is a realistic target for OCD treatment, and that continuation of SSRI protects patients against relapse. This emphasizes the importance of maintaining treatment with medication at an effective dose level in the long term, that is for at least 12 months (NICE 2006), and argues against discontinuation of treatment even after 1 year. The adage 'the dose that gets you well keeps you well' probably applies, and the possibility that some patients may retain response at a lower dose or following discontinuation must be weighed against the possibility that reinstatement of treatment after relapse may be associated with a poorer response.

Table 4.3 Double-blind studies of relapse prevention in OCD

Study	Drug	Duration prior drug treatment	n in discont. phase	Follow-up after discont.	Outcome
Bailer et al (1995)	paroxetine	6 months	44	24 weeks	Relapse rate on plac = parox parox > plac on Y-BOCS
Romano et al (1998)	fluoxetine	20 weeks	71	52 weeks	Relapse rate on plac = pooled fluox Relapse rate on plac > fluox 60mg
Koran et al (2002)	sertraline	52 weeks	223	28 weeks	Relapse rate on plac = sert Acute exacerb of OCD on plac > sert Dropout due to relapse on plac > sert
[a]Geller et al (2003)	paroxetine	16 weeks	193	16 weeks	Relapse rate on plac = parox
Hollander et al (2003)	paroxetine	12 weeks	105	36 weeks	Relapse rate on plac > parox
Fineberg et al (2006c)	escitalopram	16 weeks	322	24 weeks	Time to relapse on esc > plac Relapse rate on plac > esc

[a] in children and adolescents

> **Practice points: long-term treatment ...**
>
> • Discuss long-term medication with the patient.
> • Continue treatment for at least 12 months at the original
>   effective dose level.
> • If medication is to be discontinued, best done gradually over
>   weeks and months to mitigate possible withdrawal effects and
>   observe for signs of relapse.

4.5 Expert consensus guidelines for OCD

Expert consensus has a role in complementing and supplementing
empirical evidence. By synthesizing combined views on best practice,
a broader range of pertinent clinical questions can be addressed.
Moreover, such opinions reflect experience with a range of cases and
not just the highly selected groups that meet study criteria.

According to the Expert Consensus Panel for OCD (March et al
1997) and the World Council on Anxiety (Greist et al 2003) combined
SRI with cognitive behaviour therapy was thought the best approach
for most patients. The British Association for Psychopharmacology
(BAP) evidence-based guidelines for treating anxiety disorders, which
included OCD (Baldwin et al 2005), based its recommendations on the
level of evidence adapted from the US Agency for Health Care Policy
and Research Classification (US Department of Health and Human
Services 1992). The BAP guideline was less certain that combination
treatment was superior to psychological or serotonergic drugs given
alone. NICE consulted widely over the scope of the guideline. Published and unpublished evidence supporting the efficacy of all therapies
for OCD (and body dysmorphic disorder) were subjected to a meta-
analysis wherever possible (NICE 2006). NICE emphasized the importance of better recognition of the disorder across the lifespan, and the
need for good information and education. They recommended a
'stepped care' model, with increasing intensity of integrated drug and
psychological treatment according to clinical severity and complexity
(Box 4.2). The Canadian guidelines (June, 2006), the American Psychiatric Association guidelines and the Cape Town consensus (Zohar et al
2007) are consistent.

Box 4.2 U/S

- Awarz, J.S. (1997). Effectiveness of psychological and pharmacologi-
- Actments for obsessive compulsive disorder: a quantitative review.
- *nsult. Clin. Psychol.*, **65**: 44–52.

.erman, D.L., Greenland, S. (2002). Multivariate meta-analysis of controlled drug studies for obsessive compulsive disorder. *J. Clin. Psychopharmacol.*, **22**: 309–317.

Aizenberg, D., Naor, S., Zemishlany, Z., Weizman, A. (1999). The serotonin antagonist mianserin for treatment of serotonin-reuptake inhibitor-induced sexual dysfunction: an open-label study. *Clin. Neuropharmacol.*, **22**: 347–350.

Bairy, K.L., Madhyastha, S., Ashok, K.P., et al. (2007). Developmental and behavioral consequences of prenatal fluoxetine. *Pharmacology.*, **79**(1): 1–11.

Baldwin, D.S., Anderson, I.M., Nutt, D.J., et al. (2005). Evidence-based guidelines for the pharmacological treatment of anxiety disorders: recommendations from the British Association for Psychopharmacology. *J. Psychopharmacol.*, **19**: 567–596.

Bejerot, S., Bodlund, O. (1998). response to high doses of citalopram in treatment-resistant obsessive compulsive disorder *Acta Psychopharmacol. Scand.*, **98**: 423–424.

Bergeron, R., Ravindran, A.V., Chaput, Y., et al. (2001). Sertraline and fluoxetine treatment of obsessive compulsive disorder: results of a double-blind, 6-month treatment study. *J. Clin. Psychopharmaco.*, **22**: 148–154.

Bisserbe, J.C., Lane, R.M., Flament, M.F. (1997) A double-blind comparison of sertraline and clomipramine in outpatients with obsessive-compulsive disorder. *Euro. Psychiat.*, **12**: 82–93.

Bloch, M.H., Landeros-Weisenberger, A., Kelmendi, B., et al. (2006). Poster presented at ACNP.

Bogetto, F., Albert, U., Maina, G. (2002). Sertraline treatment of obsessive-compulsive disorder: efficacy and tolerability of a rapid titration regimen. *Euro. Neuropsychopharmacol.*, **12**: 181–186.

Byerly, M.J., Goodman, W.K., Christenen, R. (1996). High doses of sertraline for treatment-resistant obsessive compulsive disorder. *Am. J. Psychiat.*, **153**: 1232–1233.

Bystrtitsky, A., Ackerman, D.L., Rosen, R.M., et al. (2004). Augmentation of serotonin re-uptake inhibitors in refractory obsessive-compulsive disorder using adjunctive olanzapine: a placebo-controlled trial. *J. Clin. Psychiatry.*, **65**(4): 565–8.

Chouinard, G., Goodman, W., Greist, J., et al. (1990). Results of a double-blind placebo-controlled trial of a new serotonin re-uptake inhibitor, sertraline, in the treatment of obsessive-compulsive disorder. *Psychopharmaco. Bul.*, **26**: 279–284.

Clomipramine Collaborative Study Group (1991). Clomipramine in the treatment of patients with obsessive compulsive disorder. *Archs. Gen. Psychiat.*, **48**: 730–738.

Coric, V., Taskiran, S., Pittenger, C., et al. (2005 Sep 1). Riluzole augmentation in treatment-resistant obsessive-compulsive disorder: an open-label trial. *Biol. Psychiatry*, **58**(5): 424–8.

Cottraux, J., Mollard, E., Bouvard, M., et al. (1990). A controlled study of fluvoxamine and exposure in obsessive-compulsive disorder. *Int. Clin. Psychopharmacol.*, **5**: 17–30.

De Veaugh-Geiss, J., Landau, P., Katz, R. (1989). Treatment of obsessive compulsive disorder with clomipramine. *Psychiat., Ann.*, **19**: 97–101.

De Veaugh-Geiss, J., Moroz, G., Biederman, J., et al. (1992). Clomipramine hydrochloride in childhood and adolescent obsessive compulsive disorder: a multicenter trial. *J. Am. Acad. Child Adolesc. Psychiat.*, **31**: 45–49.

Fallon, B.A., Liebowitz, M.R., Campeas, R., et al. (1998). Intravenous clomipramine for obsessive-compulsive disorder refractory to oral clomipramine: a placebo-controlled study. *Archs. Gen. Psychiat.*, **55**: 918–924.

Fineberg, N.A., Roberts, A., Montgomery, S.A., Cowen, P.H. (1997). Brain 5-HT function in obsessive-compulsive disorder: prolactin responses to d-fenfluramine. *Br. J. Psychiat.*, **171**: 280–282.

Fineberg, N.A., Sivakumaran, T., Roberts, A., Gale, T. (2005). Adding quetiapine to SRI in treatment resistant obsessive compulsive disorder: a randomized controlled treatment study. *Int. Clin. Psychopharmacol.*, **20**: 223–226.

Fineberg, N., Heyman, I., Jenkins, R., et al. (2004). Does childhood and adult obsessive compulsive disorder (OCD) respond the same way to treatment with serotonin reuptake inhibitors (SRIs)? *Eur. Neuropsychopharmacol.*, **14** (Suppl. 3): S191.

Fineberg, N.A., Gale, T. (2005). Evidence-based pharmacological treatments for obsessive compulsive disorder. *Int. J. Neuropsychopharmacol.*, **8**: 107–129 (2005).

Fineberg, N.A., Stein, D.J., Premkumar, P., et al. (2006a). Adjunctive quetiapine for SRI-resistant obsessive compulsive disorder: a meta-analysis of randomised controlled treatment trials. *Int. Clin. Psychopharmacol.*, **21**: 337–343.

Fineberg, N.A., Gale, T., Sivakumaran, T. (2006b). A Review of antipsychotics in treatment resistant obsessive compulsive disorder (OCD) *J. Psychopharmacol.*, **20**: 97–103.

Fineberg, N., Lemming, O., Tonnoir, B., Stein, D.J. (2006c). Escitalopram in relapse prevention in patients with obsessive-compulsive disorder (OCD) *Eur. Neuropsychopharmacol.*, **16** (Suppl. 4): S292.

Freeman, C.P., Trimble, M.R., Deakin, J.F., et al. (1994). Fluvoxamine versus clomipramine in the treatment of obsessive-compulsive disorder: a multicenter, randomized, double-blind, parallel group comparison *J. Clin. Psychiatry*, **55**(7): 301–5.

Geller, D.A., Hoog, S.L., Heiligenstein, J.H., et al. (2001). Fluoxetine treatment for obsessive-compulsive disorder in children and Adolescents: a placebo-controlled *Clin.* trial *J. Am. Acad. Child Adolesc. Psychiat.*, **40**: 773–779.

Geller, D.A., Biederman, J., Stewart, S.E., *et al.* (2003a). Which SSRI? A meta-analysis of pharmacotherapy trials in paediatric obsessive-compulsive disorder. *Am. J. Psychiat.*, **160**: 1919–1928.

Geller, D.A., Biederman, J., Stewart, S.E., *et al.* (2003b). Impact of comorbidity on treatment response to paroxetine in paediatric obsessive compulsive disorder: is the use of exclusion criteria empirically supported in randomised controlled trials? *J. Child Adolesc. Psychopharmacol.*, **13** (Suppl.): S19–29.

Geller, D.A., Wagner, K.D., Emslie, G., Murphy, T., Carpenter, D.J., Wetherhold, E., Perera, P., machin, A., Gardiner, C., *et al.* (2004). Paroxetine treatment in children and adolescents with obsessive-compulsive disorder: a randomized, multicenter, double-blind, placebo-controlled trial. *J. Am. Acad. Child Adolesc. Psychiat.*, **43**: 1387–1396.

Goodman, W.K., Price, L.H., Rasmussen, S.A., *et al.* (1989). Efficacy of fluvoxamine in obsessive-compulsive disorder. A double-blind comparison with placebo. *Archs. Gen. Psychiat.*, **46**: 36–44.

Goodman, W.K., Kozak, M.J., Liebowitz, M., White, K.L. (1996). Treatment of obsessive-compulsive disorder with Fluvoxamine: a multicentre, double-blind, placebo-controlled trial. *Int. Clin. Psychopharmacol.*, **11**: 21–29.

Greist, J.H., Jefferson, J.W., Kobak, K.A., *et al.* (1995b). A one year double-blind placebo-controlled fixed dose study of sertraline in the treatment of obsessive-compulsive disorder. *Int. Clin. Psychopharmacol.*, **10**: 57–65.

Greist, J.H., Jefferson, J.W., Kobak, K.A., *et al.* (1995c). Efficacy and tolerability of serotonin transport inhibitors in obsessive-compulsive disorder: a meta-analysis. *Archs. Gen. Psychiat.*, **52**(1): 53–60.

Greist, J.H., Bandelow, B., Hollander, E., *et al.* (2003). Long-term treatment of obsessive-compulsive disorder in adults. *CNS Spectrums*, **8**: 7–16.

Hollander, E., Koran, L.M., Goodman, W.K., *et al.* (2003a). A double-blind placebo-controlled study of the efficacy and safety of controlled release fluvoxamine in patients with obsessive-compulsive disorder. *J. Clin. Psychiat.*, **64**: 640–647.

Hollander, E., Allen, A., Steiner, M., *et al.* (2003b). Acute and long-term treatment and prevention of relapse of obsessive-compulsive disorder with paroxetine. *J. Clin. Psychiat.*, **64**: 1113–1121.

Jenike, M.A., Hyman, S., Baer, L., *et al.* (1990a). A controlled trial of fluvoxamine in obsessive-compulsive disorder; implications for a serotonergic theory. *Am. J. Psychiat.*, **147**: 1209–1215.

Jenike, M.A., Baer, L., Summergrad, P., *et al.* (1990b). Sertraline in obsessive-compulsive disorder: a double-blind comparison with placebo. *Am. J. Psychiat.*, **147**: 923–928.

Jenike, M.A., Baer, L., Minichiello, W.E., *et al.* (1997). Placebo-controlled trial of fluoxetine and phenelzine for obsessive-compulsive disorder. *Am. J. Psychiat.*, **154**: 1261–1264.

Kobak, K.A., Greist, J.H., Jefferson, J.W., *et al.* (1998). Behavioural versus pharmacological treatments of obsessive compulsive disorder: a meta-analysis. *Psychopharmacol.*, **136**: 205–216.

Koran, L.M., McElroy, S.L., Davidson, J.R., et al. (1996 Apr). Fluxvoxamine versus clomipramine for obsessive-compulsive disorder: a double-blind comparison. *J. Clin. Psychopharmacol* **16**(2): 121–9.

Koran, L.M., Sallee, F.R., Pallantis, S. (1997). Rapid benefit of intravenous pulse-loading of clomipramine in obsessive compulsive disorder. *Am. J. Psychiat.*, **154**: 396–401.

Koran, L.M., Hackett, E., Rubin, A., et al. (2002). Efficacy of sertraline in the long-term treatment of obsessive-compulsive disorder. *Am. J. Psychiat.*, **159**: 89–95.

Kronig, M.H., Apter, J., Asnis, G., et al. (1999). Placebo-controlled, multi-center study of sertraline treatment for obsessive-compulsive disorder. *J. Clin. Psychopharmaco.*, **19**: 172–176.

Leibowitz, M.R., Turner, S.M., Piacentini, J. et al. (2002). Fluoxetine in children and Adolescents with OCD: a placebo-controlled trial. *J. Am. Acad. Child Adolesc. Psychiat.*, **41**: 1431–1438.

Lopez-Ibor J., Jr., Saiz, J., Cottraux, J., et al. (1996). Double-blind compari-son of fluoxetine versus clomipramine in the treatment of obsessive-compulsive disorder. *European Neuropsychopharmacology* **6**(2): 111–18.

Maina, G., Salvi, V., Bogetto, F. (2003a). Weight-gain during long-term drug treatment of obsessive compulsive disorder. *Eur. Neuopsycho-pharmacol.*, **13**(Suppl.): S357.

Maina, G., Albert, U., Ziero, S., Bogetto, F. (2003b). Antipsychotic aug-mentation for treatment-resistant obsessive compulsive disorder: what if antipsychotic is discontinued? *Int. Clin. Psychopharmacol.*, **18**(1): 23–28.

March, J.S., Frances, A., Kahn, D.A., Carpenter, D. (1997). The Expert Consensus Guideline series. Treatment of obsessive-compulsive disorder. *J. Clin. Psychiat.*, **58**(Suppl.): 1–72.

March, J.S., Biederman, J., Wolkow, R., et al. (1998). Sertraline in children and adolescents with obsessive compulsive disorder: a multicentre randomised controlled trial. *J. Am. Med. Assoc.*, **28**: 1752–1756.

March, J.S., Klee, B.J., Kremer, C.M. (2006). Treatment benefits and the risk of suicidality in multicenter randomised controlled trials of sertraline in children and adolescents. *Child Adolesc. Psychopharmacol.*, **16**(1–2): 91–102.

Milanfranchi, A., Ravagli, S., Lensi, P., et al. (1997 May). A double-blind study of fluvoxamine and clomipramine in the treatment of obsessive-compulsive disorder. *Int. Clin. Psychopharmacol.*, **12**(3): 131–6.

Monteiro, W.O., Noshirvani, H.F., Marks, I.M., Lelliott, P.T. (1987). Anor-gasmia from clomipramine in obsessive-compulsive disorder: a controlled trial. *Br. J. Psychiat.*, **151**: 107–112.

Montgomery, S.A. (1980). Clomipramine in obsessional neurosis: a placebo-controlled trial. *Pharmacol. Med.*, **1**: 189–192.

Montgomery, S.A., McIntyre, A., Osterheider, M. et al. (1993). A double-blind placebo-controlled study of fluoxetine in patients with DSM-IIIR obsessive compulsive disorder. *Eur. Neuropsychopharmacol.*, **3**: 143–152.

Montgomery, S.A., Kasper, S., Stein, D.J. et al. (2001). Citalopram 20mg, 40mg, and 60mg are all effective and well tolerated compared with placebo in obsessive-compulsive disorder. *Int. Clin. Psychopharmacol.*, **16**: 75–86.

Mundo, E., Bianchi, L., Bellodi, L. (1997a). Efficacy of fluvoxamine, paroxetine, and citalopram in the treatment of obsessive-compulsive disorder; a single-blind study. *J. Clin. Psychopharmacol.*, **17**: 267–71.

NICE 2006: Obsessive-compulsive disorder: Core interventions in the treatment of obsessive-compulsive disorder and body-dysmorphic disorder. National Collaborating Centre for Mental Health, Publ. British Psychological Society and the Royal College of Psychiatrists, UK, 2006. Also at www.nice.org.uk.

Pallanti, S., Querciolil, L., Paiva, R.S., et al. (1999). Citalopram for treatment-resistant obsessive-compulsive disorder. *European Psychiatry*, **14**: 101–6.

Pediatric OCD Treatment Study (POTS) team. (2004). Cognitive-behavior therapy, sertraline, and their combination for children and Adolescents with obsessive-compulsive disorder: the Pediatric OCD Treatment Study (POTS) randomized controlled trial. *J. Am. Med. Assoc.*, **292**: 1969–1976.

Perse, T., Greist, J.H., Jefferson, J.W., et al. (1987). Fluvoxamine treatment of obsessive compulsive disorder. *Am. J. Psychiat.*, **144**: 1543–1548.

Piccinelli, M., Pini, S., Bellantuono, C., Wilkinson, G. (1995). Efficacy of drug treatment in obsessive compulsive disorder. *Br. J. Psychiat.*, **166**: 424–443.

Pigott, T.A., Pato, M.T., Bernstein, S.E., et al. (1990 Oct). Controlled comparisons of clomipramine and fluoxetine in the treatment of obsessive-compulsive disorder. Behavioral and biological results. *Arch. Gen. Psychiatry.*, **47**(10): 926–32.

Pigott, T.A., Seay, S.M. (1999). A review of the efficacy of selective serotonin reuptake inhibitors in obsessive compulsive disorder. *J. Clin. Psychiat.*, **60**: 101–106.

Poyurovsky, M., Weizman, R., Weizman, A., et al. (2005 Nov). Memantine for treatment-resistant OCD. *Am. J. Psychiatry.*, **162**(11): 2191–2.

Rasmussen, S., Hackett, E., Duboff, E., et al. (1997). A 2-year study of sertraline in the treatment of obsessive-compulsive disorder. *Int. Clin. Psychopharmacol.*, **12**: 309–316.

Riddle, M.A., Scahill, L., King, R.A., et al. (1992). Double-blind crossover trial of fluoxetine and placebo in children and Adolescents with obsessive compulsive disorder. *J. Am. Acad. Child Adolesc. Psychiat.*, **31**: 1062–1069.

Riddle, M.A., Reeve, E.A., Yaryura-Tobias, J., et al. (2001). Fluvoxamine for children and adolescents with obsessive compulsive disorder; a randomised, controlled multicentre trial. *J. Am. Acad. of Child Adolesc. Psychiat.*, **40**: 222–229.

Romano, S., Goodman, W.K., Tamura, R., et al. (2001). Long-term treatment of obsessive-compulsive disorder after an acute response: a comparison of fluoxetine versus placebo. *J. Clin. Psychopharmacol.*, **21**: 46–52.

Rouillon, F. (1998). A double-blind comparison of fluvoxamine and clomipramine in OCD. *Eur. Neuropsychopharmacol.,* **8**(Suppl.): 260–261.

Shapira, N.A., Ward, H.E., Mandoki, M., *et al.* (2004). A double blind placebo-controlled trial of olanzapine in fluoxetine-refractory obsessive-compulsive disorder. *Biol. Psychiat.,* **55**: 553–63.

Sheehan, D.V., Harnett-Sheehan, K., Raj, B.A. (1996). The measurement of disability. *Int. Clin. Psychopharmacol.,* **11**(Suppl.): 89–95.

Simpson, H.B., Huppert, J.D., Petkova, E., *et al.* (2006). Response versus remission in obsessive compulsive disorder. J. Clin. *Psychiat.,* **67**: 269–276.

Smeraldi, E., Erzegovesi, S., Bianchi, I. (1992) Fluvoxamine versus clomipramine treatment in obsessive-compulsive disorder: a preliminary study. *New Trends in Experimental and Clinical Psychiatry.,* **8**: 63–65.

Stein, D.J., Spadaccini, F., Hollander, E. (1995). Meta-analysis of pharmacotherapy trials of obsessive compulsive disorder. *Int. Clin. Psychopharmacol.,* **10**: 11–18.

Stein, D.J., Tonnoir, B., Andersen, E.W., Fineberg, N. (2007). *Eur. Neuropsychopharmacol.,* **16**(Suppl. 4): S295.

Szegedi, A., Wetzel, H., Leal, M., *et al.* (1996). Combination treatment with clomipramine and fluvoxamine: drug monitoring, safety and tolerability data. *J. Clin. Psychiat.,* **57**: 257–264.

Tenney, N.H., Denys, D.A., Van Megen, H.J.G.M., *et al.* (2003). Effect of a pharmacological intervention on quality of life in patients with obsessive-compulsive disorder. *Int. Clin. Psychopharmacol.,* **18**: 29–33.

Tollefson, G., Rampey, A., Potvin, J., *et al.* (1994) A multicenter investigation of fixed-dose fluoxetine in the treatment of obsessive compulsive disorder. *Archs. Gen. Psychiat.,* **51**: 559–567.

Wilens, T.E., Biederman, J., March, J., *et al.* (1999). Absence of cardiovascular and adverse effects of sertraline in children and Adolescents. *J. Am. Acad. Child Adolesc. Psychiat.,* **38**: 573–577.

Zohar, J., Judge, R. (1996). Paroxetine versus clomipramine in the treatment of obsessive compulsive disorder. *Br. J. Psychiat.,* **169**: 468–474.

Zohar, J., Hollander, E., Stein, D.J., *et al.* (2007). *CNS Spectrums,* **2**(suppl. 3), 59–63.

Chapter 5

Psychotherapy: an integrated approach

Key points

- Behavioural therapy is effective in both adult and paediatric OCD
- Exposure therapy is a key component of behavioural therapy
- Cognitive interventions may also play a role in the treatment of OCD
- It is useful to obtain a patient's explanatory model of their disorder
- Both pharmacotherapy and psychotherapy reverse striatal dysfunction in OCD

5.1 Introduction

In this chapter we provide a brief introduction to the different types of psychotherapy for obsessive-compulsive disorder (OCD). We then focus on the question of how to conceptualize and implement an integrated approach to the management of OCD. We do this by attempting to define the core psychobiological deficit in OCD, and then considering how both pharmacotherapy and psychotherapy can reverse this dysfunction. Readers who are interested in more detail on the specific techniques employed in cognitive-behavioural therapy (CBT) of OCD, are referred to more specialized texts (see Chapter 7).

5.2 Psychotherapies for OCD

Psychoanalytic treatment for obsessive-compulsive neurosis was described by Freud, and was subsequently long thought to be an effective approach to management (Stein & Stone 1997). However, despite the contribution of psychodynamic authors to delineating the phenomenology and psychology of OCD, there is insufficient evidence to support the current use of psychoanalytic treatment for this condition (NICE 2005).

Behavioural therapy was the first psychotherapy for which careful empirical support was obtained (Marks 1997). It is useful in both adult and paediatric OCD (Greist 1994; March et al. 2001). A particularly important component of behavioural therapy appears to be exposure to the feared stimuli. The precise way in which exposure results in normalization of cortico-striatal-thalamic cortical (CSTC) circuitry remains, however, to be fully understood.

In behavioural therapy, a hierarchy of feared situations is created, and the patient then practises facing the fear (exposure), while monitoring the anxiety and experiencing that it lessens without the need to carry out a ritual (response prevention). It is crucial to begin by educating the patient about the way in which the therapy works, and to then engage the patient by using a graded programme and collaboratively tackling the easiest challenges first. Homework practice is also a crucial part of the therapy.

There may also be a role for cognitive interventions in the treatment of OCD (Salkovskis 1999). Several belief domains are likely to be important in OCD, including inflated responsibility; overimportance of thoughts; excessive concern about the importance of controlling one's thoughts; and overestimation of threat (Obsessive Compulsive Cognitions Working Group 1997). These kinds of faulty reasoning are able to serve as targets in the cognitive therapy.

Cognitive approaches encourage patients to re-evaluate overvalued beliefs, to regain a more realistic perspective on the importance of their thoughts, and to carry out 'behavioural experiments' to test the validity of their beliefs about control and about threat. Cognitive approaches may be as effective as exposure procedures, but it is not clear whether the addition of cognitive techniques significantly improves the efficacy of exposure and response prevention (Abramowitz 1997; NICE 2005).

In practice, however, given that exposure and response prevention (ERP) may require some change in cognition prior to its use, there is an overlap between these approaches, and in clinical settings a 'cognitive-behavioural' approach is often used, administered individually or in groups, with the contexts ranging from self-help computer instruction through to intensive hospitalization (Thornicroft et al 1991; Bachofen et al 1999). Given that there may be significant family accommodation to OCD symptoms, assessing such accommodation and including the patient's partner or family in developing a treatment strategy is appropriate in some cases, particularly children and adolescents with OCD (Calvocoressi et al 1999).

There is unfortunately relatively little empirical data addressing the question of how best to sequence or combine pharmacotherapy and psychotherapy from OCD. Nevertheless, from a theoretical viewpoint, there may be value in integrating different modalities

(Stein et al 2001). In clinical practice it would seem sensible to encourage patients who are on medication also to understand and adhere to the principles of CBT, and a number of studies support the value of adding a CBT intervention to OCD patients on medication (O'Connor et al 1999; Simpson et al 1999).

5.3 What is the core psychobiological deficit in OCD?

An integrated approach to the treatment of OCD would ideally rest on the basis of a clear understanding of the nature of the core psychobiological deficit underlying the disorder. Despite significant neurobiological advances in the field, defining a core psychobiological deficit in OCD remains an ambitious undertaking. As a first step towards this goal, we would tentatively suggest that the fundamental deficiency in OCD revolves around faults in the selection, maintenance and termination of 'procedural strategies', particularly (but not exclusively) those involving harm assessment.

This characterization requires some explanation. We can begin by recalling that the bulk of current evidence – neuropsychological, neuro-imaging, neuro-immunological, and neurosurgical – emphasizes the role of CSTC dysfunction in OCD (Rauch & Baxter 1998; Stein et al 2000; Whiteside et al 2004). The immediate question, then, is what is the normal role of these circuits? From there, it might be possible to determine the nature of the core dysfunction in OCD.

It is widely believed that CTSC circuits play a role in organizing motor and cognitive procedural strategies (Robins & Brown 1990; Cummings 1993; Saint-Cyr et al 1995). Take, for example, the procedure for riding a bicycle. When we initially learn to ride, the effort requires a good deal of conscious concentration. However, over time, the brain-mind encodes a 'bicycling procedure' – this procedure is enacted non-consciously and automatically under the direction of the striatum. Even when we lose our explicit memories of learning to ride a bicycle, our implicit knowledge of how to ride remains (this kind of dissociation has been documented, for example, in studies of dementia).

There is evidence suggesting that the neural mechanisms underlying procedural knowledge are disrupted in OCD, with evidence of disinhibition (Chamberlain et al 2005). For example, when undertaking an implicit cognition task during functional brain imaging, normal controls demonstrated activation of CSTC circuits (especially striatum), but OCD patients showed a pathological activation of temporal regions instead (Rauch et al 1997). Of course, OCD is not a dysfunction in bicycling; rather, OCD typically involves those procedures that involve the assessment of harm. Thus, although OCD has been suggested to be a disorder of grooming (and some associated symptoms, such as tics, are primarily motoric), in patients with cleaning rituals there are invariably concerns about the harm of contamination.

The fact that the orbitofrontal cortex rather than the amygdala is predominantly activated in brain-imaging studies of OCD suggests that the stimuli which generate anxiety for the OCD sufferer originate internally rather than externally. In contrast, in post-traumatic stress disorder (PTSD) a loud noise may stimulate thalamo-amygdaloid activation and produce an implicit, automatic fear response (startle reaction, etc.). It is hypothesized that in OCD, once a trigger – say a speck of dirt – has been noticed, an internal cognitive process, perhaps comprising disrupted or inefficient striatal processing, results in the exaggeration of its potential harmful consequences.

5.4 Core deficit versus compensatory dysfunctions

Although it is possible that increased orbito-frontal activation represents a primary lesion in OCD, there is increasing support for the idea that it is instead a compensatory response. In this view, orbito-frontal activation represents a compensatory reaction to dysfunction in subcortical structures, along the lines of a 'natural defence' against obsessional anxiety. Thus, increased activity in orbito-frontal cortex may be an attempt to suppress striatally mediated harm exaggeration in OCD. It has been suggested that one of the roles of treatment may be to bolster this 'natural defence' mechanism.

The finding that OCD patients with low orbito-frontal activity prior to treatment are less likely to respond to medication (Swedo et al 1992), is in line with this hypothesis. It is as if there is not enough capacity in the system for adequate compensation to be achieved. Similarly, it is interesting that the behavioural exacerbation of OCD by sumatriptan, a specific agonist of the terminal autoreceptor ($5-HT_{1B/D}$), appears to be associated with decreased activity in areas of prefrontal cortex (Stein et al 1999), perhaps suggesting that the level of activity in the compensatory circuitry has been turned down by the drug.

It is notable that certain serotonergic systems appear underactive in untreated OCD [e.g. blunted prolactin response to the serotonergic agonist m-chlorophenylpiperazine (m-CPP)] (Zohar et al 1987; Hollander et al 1992) as well as in impulsivity (Stein et al 1993). The cognitive process whereby a speck of dirt triggers exaggerated fear of harm (by contamination) and sets off hand-washing compulsions may well reflect striatal serotonergic hypofunction. Conversely, there is also evidence of hyperserotonergic function in OCD (e.g. enhanced growth hormone responses to l-tryptophan and d-fenfluramine)

(Fineberg et al 1994, 1997), symptom exacerbation after m-CPP (Hollander et al 1992; Zohar et al 1997), and this may represent prefrontal compensatory mechanisms at work.

This view of underlying deficit and secondary compensation in OCD provides a speculative way of tying together a range of neuro-anatomical and neurochemical findings. But does it make sense in terms of our clinical understanding of the symptomatology and experience of suffering from OCD?

One of the most convincing descriptions of the phenomenology of OCD turns out to be that of Freud. Indeed, Freud's understanding of obsessional neurosis provides a cornerstone for psychodynamic theory, and is consistent with much modern thinking about the operation of an unconscious. For Freud, at the heart of obsessional neurosis are unconscious aggressive instincts (Freud, 1926). Unaccept-able urges, particularly hostile urges, are admitted into awareness because of incomplete repression, necessitating defensive responses in the form of compulsive rituals to reduce guilt and anxiety.

This formulation is redolent of the psychobiological characteriza-tion above. In OCD there may be a non-conscious, striatally-mediated impulsive/disinhibited process. This results in frontally mediated com-pensatory attempts to switch this process off. A range of more recent data support a link between OCD and behavioural disinhibition. Epidemiological data indicate that OCD is frequently associated with a history of childhood impulsivity and aggression (Hollander et al 1997). Furthermore, in clinical settings, individuals with OCD often demonstrate a degree of impulsive aggression (Stein & Hollander 1993), which, given their harm avoidance, is counter-intuitively high.

So far we have concentrated on the central theme of harm assessment in OCD. Other authors (e.g. Tallis 1995) have drawn attention to the role of doubt in this disorder. According to Freud, doubt leads the patient to uncertainty about his protective measures, and to his continual repetition of them in order to banish that uncer-tainty. It is as though obsessional patients have lost the ability to register they have done something, or even to 'know if they know something' (Rapoport, 1989).

It has been suggested that dysfunction of CSTC circuits may inter-fere with the normal verification of the successful completion of preventive or reparative behaviours, leading to compulsive repetition of the behaviours until appropriate information processing is accom-plished (Stein & Hollander 1992; Szechtman et al 2004). Just how the compulsion eventually stops is not clear; perhaps the energy dissipates a little like that of a tuning fork.

5.5 **An integrated approach to treatment**

If the core psychobiological dysfunction in OCD revolves around striatally mediated problems in the selection, maintenance and termination of procedural strategies, how might we approach treatment?

First, serotonergic medication can be used to optimize striatal function, either by direct actions at receptors in the striatum, or by augmenting orbito-striatal compensatory mechanisms, as described above. Where striatal damage is more extensive, dopamine blockers may provide an additional mechanism for increased serotonergic neuronal activity, since dopaminergic neurons act to inhibit striatal serotonergic neurons (McDougle et al 2000; Fineberg & Gale 2005).

Second, cognitive-behavioural techniques can be used to regulate striatal function. For some reason, exposure to feared stimuli, such as pharmacotherapy, ultimately results in optimization of the CTSC circuits. Baxter's elegant work showing comparable effects of an selective serotonin reuptake inhibitor (SSRI) and behavioural therapy on the functional neuroanatomy of OCD remains a key support for the idea of an integrated brain-mind approach to OCD (Baxter et al 1992). Subsequent studies have consolidated and expanded this early work (Benazon et al 2003).

Third, there may be a range of preventative interventions that can be applied, early in life, to protect the striatum. The basal ganglia are particularly vulnerable to neonatal hypoxaemia, and preventing this is therefore important. The finding that childhood emotional deprivation is associated with neuro-anatomical abnormalities in the striatum (Martin et al 1991) provides an even more challenging area for therapeutic intervention.

Finally, auto-immune processes in the aftermath of infection with streptococcus may also result in striatal damage (Swedo et al 1998). It will be interesting to see whether prophylactic measures including aggressive early diagnosis and intervention with antibiotics are ultimately able to have a postive impact on the occurrence and course of paediatric auto-immune neuropsychiatric disorders (PANDAS) (Swedo & Grant, 2005).

5.6 **Are integrated treatments more effective in OCD?**

We know that SRIs and behaviour therapy are individually effective in OCD, and it would therefore seem likely that the combination of both treatments would provide even better efficacy. In fact, there have been few studies looking at this area, and the evidence to date remains incomplete (Fineberg et al 1997b; NICE 2005). Meta-analyses (e.g. Picinelli et al 1995) have not succeeded in addressing the question of relative efficacy of interventions, partly because this kind of statistical approach cannot adequately correct for the changes that have occurred between individual trials over the years (e.g. rising placebo-response rates over the past 10 years, greater numbers of treatment-resistant and atypical patients entering later medication trials (see Chapter 4)). Head-to-head comparisons of the effects of combination treatment compared with drug or behavioural monotherapy are preferable, and it is regrettable that so few properly controlled studies have been performed.

Early influential studies by Marks et al (1980, 1988) were the first to address the question of how best to sequence and combine pharmacotherapy and psychotherapy in OCD. Their first study suggested that the addition of clomipramine to behaviour therapy enhanced compliance and produced a more favourable outcome (Marks et al 1980). These results were echoed in the second study, where the addition of clomipramine to exposure therapy produced a greater level of improvement (Marks et al 1988). Unfortunately these studies are limited by a number of methodological problems including the use of rather small sample sizes.

Two small studies (Cottraux et al 1990; Hohagen et al 1997) compared fluvoxamine plus behaviour therapy with placebo plus behaviour therapy, and, in spite of small numbers, demonstrated superior efficacy for the combination over exposure monotherapy for up to 6 months. There was no drug monotherapy arm in one of the studies (Hohagen et al 1997). The study by Cottraux et al (1990) was unable to show a significant advantage for combined drug and exposure compared with fluvoxamine, even though the drug was given in combination with anti-exposure instructions (which should have had an adverse effect), but the study was probably underpowered ($n = 40$), and the authors themselves advocated further, larger studies.

However, subsequent trials, even when undertaken with a larger sample, have remained unable to confirm the benefit of combining pharmacotherapy with psychotherapy. In a recent trial in children and adolescents with OCD, placebo pill was compared with sertraline alone, CBT alone, and CBT plus sertraline (March et al 2006). All three active treatments were better than placebo, but they did not differ significantly from one another. Optimistic claims from uncontrolled case-series that CBT prevents relapse if medication is prematurely discontinued (e.g. March et al 1994), although intuitively persuasive, need to be explored further under properly controlled conditions.

powerful model of a contemporary approach to the brain-mind, to psychopathology, and to treatment. In the clinical setting it is useful to be able to educate the patient that the 'false alarm' in their brain-mind can be reset through a combination of pharmacotherapy and exposure. For researchers, determining the precise mechanisms through which these interventions operate remains an exciting challenge for the future.

References

NICE Clinical Guideline 31. Obsessive-Compulsive Disorder: Core interventions in the treatment of obsessive-compulsive disorder and body dysmorphic disorder. www.nice.org.uk. 2005.

NICE 2006: Obsessive-compulsive disorder: Core interventions in the treatment of obsessive-compulsive disorder and body-dysmorphic disorder. National Collaborating Centre for Mental Health, Publ., British Psychological Society and the Royal College of Psychiatrists, UK, 2006. Also at www.NICE.org.uk

Abramowitz, J.S. (1997). Effectiveness of psychological and pharmacological treatments for obsessive-compulsive disorder: a quantitative review. *J. Consult. Clin. Psychol.*, **65**: 44–52.

Bachofen, M., Nakagawa, A., Marks, I.M., et al. (1999). Home self-assessment and self-treatment of obsessive-compulsive disorder using a manual and a computer-conducted telephone interview: replication of a UK–US study. *J. Clin. Psychiat.*, **60**: 545–549.

Baxter, L.R., Schwartz, J.M., Bergman, K.S., et al. (1992). Caudate glucose metabolic rate changes with both drug and behaviour therapy for OCD. *Arch. Gen. Psychiatry.*, **49**: 681–689.

Benazon, N.R., Moore, G.J., Rosenberg, D.R. (2003). Neurochemical analyses in pediatric obsessive-compulsive disorder in patients treated with cognitive-behavioural therapy. *J. Am. Acad. Child Adolesc. Psychiat.*, **42**, 1279–1285.

Bystritsky, A., Munford, P.R., Rosen, R.M., et al. (1996). A preliminary study of partial hospital management of severe obsessive-compulsive disorder. *Psychiat. Serv.*, **47**:170–174.

Calvocoressi, L., Mazure, C.M., Kasl, S., et al. (1999). Family accommodation of obsessive-compulsive symptoms: instrument development and assessment of family behavior. *J. Nerv. Ment. Dis.*, **187**: 636–642.

Chamberlain, S.R., Blackwell, A.D., Fineberg, N.A., et al. (2005). The neuropsychology of obsessive compulsive disorder: the importance of failures in cognitive and behavioural inhibition as candidate endophenotypic markers. *Neurosci. Biobehav. Rev.*, **29**: 399–419.

Cottraux, J., Mollard, E., Bouvard, M., et al. (1990). A controlled study of fluvoxamine and exposure in obsessive-compulsive disorder. *Int. Clin. Psychopharmacol.*, **5**: 17–30.

Cummings, J.L. (1993). Frontal-subcortical circuits and human behaviour. *Arch. Neurol.*, **50**: 873–880.

Fineberg, N.A., Gale, T.M. (2005). Evidence-based pharmacotherapy of obsessive-compulsive disorder. *Int. J. Neuropsychopharmacol.*, **8**: 107–129.

Freud, S. (1926). *Inhibitions, symptoms, and anxiety.* Standard Edition., **20**: 111–131.

Garvey, M.A., Perlmutter, S.A., Allen, A.J., *et al.* (1999). A pilot study of penicillin prophylaxis for neuropsychiatric exacerbations triggered by streptococcal infections. *Biol. Psychiatry*, **45**: 1564–1571.

Greist, J.H. (1994). Behavior therapy for obsessive compulsive disorder. *J. Clin. Psychiat.*, **55** (Suppl): 60–68.

Hohagen, F., Winkelmann, G., Rasche-Rauchle, H., *et al.*, (1998). Combination of behaviour therapy with fluvoxamine in comparison with behaviour therapy and placebo: results of a multi-centre study. *Brit. Jnl. Psychiatry*, **173** (suppl. 35), 71–78.

Hollander, E., DeCaria, C., Nitescu, A., *et al.* (1992). Serotonergic function in obsessive-compulsive disorder: Behavioural and neuroendocrine responses to oral m-CPP and fenfluramine in patients and healthy volunteers. *Arch. Gen. Psychiatry*, **49**: 21–28.

March, J.S., Mulle, K., Herbel, B. (1994). Behavioural psychotherapy for children and adolescents with obsessive-compulsive disorder: an open trial of a new protocol driven treatment package. *J. Am. Acad. Child Adolesc. Psychiatry*, **33**: 333–41.

March, J.S., Franklin, M., Nelson, A., Foa, E. (2001). Cognitive-behavioural psychotherapy for pediatric obsessive-compulsive disorder. *J. Clin. Child. Psychol.*, **30**: 8–18.

March, J.S., Klee, B.J., Kremer, C.M. (2006). Treatment benefits and the risk of suicidality in multi-centre randomised controlled trials of sertraline in children and adolescents. *Child Adolsc. Psychopharmacol.*, **16** (1–2): 91–102.

Marks, I.M., Stern, R.S., Mawson, D., *et al.* (1980). Clomipramine and exposure for obsessive-compulsive rituals. *I. Br. J. Psychiatry*, **136**: 1–25.

Marks, I.M., Lelliott, P., Basoglu, M., *et al.* (1988). Clomipramine, self exposure and therapist aided exposure for obsessive-compulsive rituals. *Br. J. Psychiatry*, **152**: 522–534.

Marks, I. (1997). Behaviour therapy for obsessive-compulsive disorder: a decade of progress. *Can. J. Psychiat.*, **42**: 1021–1027.

Martin, L.J., Spicer, D.M., Lewis, M.H., *et al.* (1991) Social deprivation of infant monkeys alters the chemoarchitecture of the brain: I. Subcortical regions. *J. Neurosci.*, **11**: 3344–3358.

McDougle, C.J., Goodman, W.K., Leckman, J.F., *et al.* (1994). Haloperidol addition in fluvoxamine-refractory obsessive-compulsive disorder: A double-blind placebo-controlled study in patients with and without tics. *Arch. Gen. Psychiatry*, **51**. 302–308.

O'Connor, K., Todorov, C., Robillard, S. *et al.* (1999) Cognitive-behaviour therapy and medication in the treatment of obsessive-compulsive disorder: a controlled study. *Can. J. Psychiat.* **44**: 64–71.

Obsessive Compulsive Cognitions Working Group (1997). Cognitive assessment of obsessive-compulsive disorder. *Behav. Res. Ther.*, **35**: 667–681.

Picinelli, M., Pini, S., Bellatuono, C., et al. (1995). Efficacy of drug treatment in obsessive-compulsive disorder: A meta-analytic review. Brit. J. Psychiatry, **166**: 424–443.

Rapoport, J.L. (1989). The boy who couldn't stop washing: The experience and treatment of obsessive-compulsive disorder. E.P. Dutton, New York.

Rauch, S.L., Baxter, L.R. Jr. Neuroimaging in obsessive-compulsive disorder and related disorders: In Jenicke, M.A., Baer, L., Minichiello, W.E. (eds) (1998). Obsessive-Compulsive Disorders: Practical Management. 3rd ed. Mosby, St. Louis.

Rauch, S.L., Savage, C.R., Alpert, N.M., et al. (1997). Probing striatal function in obsessive-compulsive disorder: A PET study of implicit sequence learning. J. Neuropsychiatry, **9**: 568–573.

Robbins, T.W., Brown, V.J. (1990). The role of the striatum in the mental chronometry of action: a theoretical review. Rev. Neurosci., **2**: 181–213.

Saint-Cyr, J.A., Taylor, A.E., Nicholson, K. Behaviour and the basal ganglia. In: Weiner, W.J., Lang, A.E. (eds) (1995). Behavioural Neurology of Movement Disorders. Raven Press, New York.

Salkovskis, P.M. (1999). Understanding and treating obsessive-compulsive disorder. Behav. Res. Ther., **37**(suppl): 29–52.

Simpson, H.B., Gorinkle, K.S., Liebowitz, M.R. (1999). Cognitive-behavioural therapy as an adjunct to serotonin reuptake inhibitors in obsessive-compulsive disorder: an open trial. J. Clin. Psychiat., **60**: 584–590.

Stein, D.J., Hollander, E. (1993). Impulsive aggression and obsessive-compulsive disorder. Psychiatric Annals, **23**:389–395.

Stein, D.J., Rapoport, J.L. (1996). Cross-cultural studies and obsessive-compulsive disorder. CNS Spectrums, **1**: 42–46.

Stein, D.J., Fineberg, N., Seedat, S. (2001). An integrated approach to the treatment of OCD. In Fineberg, N., Marazziti, D., and Stein, D.J. eds, Obsessive-Compulsive Disorder: A Practical Guide., Martin Seedat, London.

Stein, D.J., Stone, M.H. (1997). Essential Papers on Obsessive-Compulsive Disorders. New York University Press, New York.

Swedo, S.E., Leonard, H.L., Rapoport, J.L. (2004). The pediatric autoimmune neuropsychiatric disorders associated with streptococcal infection (PANDAS) subgroup: separating fact from fiction. Pediatrics, **113**: 907–911.

Swedo, S.E., Grant, P.J. (2005). Annotation: PANDAS: A model for human autoimmune disease. J. Child Psychol. Psychiat. Allied Discipl., **46**: 227–234.

Szechtman, H., Woody, E. (2004). Obsessive-compulsive disorder as a disturbance of security motivation. Psychol. Rev., **111**: 111–127.

Tallis, F. (1995). Obsessive-Compulsive Disorder, a Cognitive and Neuropsychological Perspective. John Wiley and Sons Ltd., UK.

Thornicroft, G., Colson, L., Marks, I. (1991). An in-patient behavioural psychotherapy unit. Description and audit. Br. J. Psychiat., **158**: 362–367.

Whiteside, S.P., Port, J.D., Abramowitz, J.S. (2004). A meta-analysis of functional neuroimaging in obsessive-compulsive disorder. Psychiat. Res., **132**: 69–79.

Zohar, J., Mueller, E.A., Insel, T.R., et al. (1987). Serotonergic responsivity in obsessive-compulsive disorder: Comparison of patients and healthy controls. Arch. Gen. Psychiatry, **44**: 946–951.

Chapter 6

Conclusion

This volume has covered the phenomenology, psychobiology, pharmacotherapy, and psychotherapy of obsessive-compulsive disorder (OCD). We have also briefly considered some of the OCD-related conditions. We have attempted to synthesize the growing research literature, with the aim of providing practical guidance to clinicians.

Significant advances have been made in describing the complex phenomenology of OCD, and this has important practical implications. First, given the high prevalence of OCD and related conditions there is growing consensus that there is value in screening patients with simple questions, such as those listed by Zohar and Fineberg. A high index of suspicion for OCD is justified in a number of contexts, including dermatology clinics, patients with tics, and pregnancy. Additional work is needed to reverse the underdiagnosis and undertreatment of OCD.

Second, there is again a good deal of consensus that only a few symptom dimensions capture much of the variance in OCD symptoms. Of course, it is important for clinicians to remain on the lookout for rarer forms of OCD. However, instruments such as the dimensional Yale–Brown Obsessive Compulsive Scale (DY-BOCS), which focus on four key symptom dimensions, appear to be useful in the clinical setting. Instruments are also available for the assessment of OCD symptoms in children and adolescents.

Third, many authors have emphasized that OCD overlaps phenomenologically and psychobiologically with conditions such as Tourette's syndrome and body dysmorphic disorder, whereas it has less in common with the anxiety disorders. Although the concept of the 'OCD spectrum' requires further research and validation, it has immediate utility in the clinical setting. In particular, patients with OCD should be screened for OCD spectrum disorders, and patients with OCD spectrum disorders typically deserve a trial of anti-OCD treatment.

In Chapter 3, on the pathogenesis of OCD, we emphasized the value of a cortico-striatal-thalamic-cortical (CSTC) model for conceptualizing the psychobiology of OCD. A focus on CSTC circuitry allows an integration of several different sets of data on OCD, ranging from cognitive and affective studies, through to brain imaging research, and on to more molecular work on this disorder. In addition, a focus on CSTC circuitry provides a basis for integrating work on the pharmacotherapy, psychotherapy, and neurosurgical treatment of OCD.

We can briefly review some of these data here. First, involvement of the CSTC circuitry in OCD is useful in understanding studies on the neuropsychiatry and neuropsychology of OCD. These have demonstrated an association between OCD and motoric symptoms (such as tics), cognitive disruptions (e.g. impairment in implicit learning), and affective dysregulation (e.g. impairments in the processing of emotion). The striatum mediates a broad range of motoric, cognitive, and affective functions, consistent with the wide range of impairments found in OCD and related conditions.

Second, involvement of the CSTC circuitry is useful in integrating data on structural, functional, and molecular imaging in OCD. Although structural findings have documented involvement of the striatum in OCD, it is possible that increased volume is seen during acute episodes of PANDAS (paediatric auto-immune neuropsychiatric disorders associated with streptococcal infection), while decreased volumes are characteristic of more chronic disease. Functional imaging studies have demonstrated increased activity at rest, and especially during symptom provocation, in CSTC circuitry. Cognitive and affective paradigms (e.g. implicit learning) also demonstrate disruption of CSTC function in OCD.

Third, there is a growing understanding of the specific molecular alterations found in CSTC circuitry, which may be associated with OCD. Genetic studies have indicated that some patients with OCD have rare functional variations in the serotonin transporter in serotonergic neurons that play a key role in the striatum. Studies of dopamine-receptor binding have also demonstrated abnormalities in basal ganglia circuitry in OCD. Magnetic resonance spectroscopy has indicated alterations in the glutamatergic system in CSTC circuitry in OCD.

Fourth, a CSTC model is useful in providing an integrated understanding of different therapeutic approaches to OCD. Pharmacotherapy, psychotherapy and neurosurgery all result in a normalization of the dysfunction in CSTC circuitry that is so characteristic of OCD. Nevertheless, it appears that pharmacotherapy and psychotherapy have different predictors of response; thus each may exert its effect in a unique way. Although the combination of pharmacotherapy and psychotherapy does not always yield a more robust response than either modality alone, there remains a theoretical rationale for using both forms of treatment together.

Finally, we have reviewed current knowledge of the pharmacotherapy and psychotherapy of OCD. Meta-analyses of the randomized controlled trials in OCD have clearly demonstrated that selective serotonin reuptake inhibitors (SSRIs) are the medication treatment of choice, while CBT (with exposure and response prevention) is the

Table 6.1 OCD spectrum disorders that may respond to SSRIs

- Body dysmorphic disorder
- Hypochondriasis
- OC symptoms in autistic disorder
- OC symptoms in mental retardation
- OC symptoms in Tourette's disorder
- Olfactory reference syndromes
- Onychophagia (severe nail biting)
- Skin-picking
- Trichotillomania

psychotherapy of choice in OCD. The efficacy of SSRIs and CBT is clear not only in adults, but also in children and adolescents with OCD.

Several consensus documents have been published on OCD. The Cape Town consensus emphasized that that SSRIs are the first choice of medication in OCD. It noted that these agents may need to be given at a higher dose, and for longer duration, than is usually the case in disorders such as depression. The SSRIs are useful not only for OCD, but also for a range of related conditions (see Table 6.1). Finally, patients with OCD not only respond to medication, some experience significant improvement in symptoms, and sometimes even remission.

In the management of refractory patients, a number of key principles must be underlined. Diagnosis should be re-considered and general medical conditions excluded. Medication history should be carefully reviewed, and adherence to medication established. Dopamine blockers are currently the pharmacotherapy augmentation strategy of choice, and should be effective in around 50% of patients. In those patients who fail to respond to a range of SSRIs and augmentation stragies, more unusual interventions can be considered (including IV clomipramine, repetitive transcranial magnetic stimulation (rTMS), deep brain stimulation and stereotactic neurosurgery). A full discussion of these techniques, however, is beyond this volume.

A final crucial component of treatment is psycho-education. Consumer advocacy groups have played a vital role in increasing awareness of this disorder in the community, and in encouraging early diagnosis and treatment. The internet provides a number of excellent resources for OCD patients, and a number of virtual support groups are useful for some patients. Additional work is needed to improve mental health literacy in general, and knowledge of OCD in particular.

Taken together, advances in understanding the phenomenology, psychobiology, pharmacotherapy, and psychotherapy of OCD have improved the prognosis of those diagnosed with OCD. Nevertheless, much remains to be learned about this intriguing and complex disorder. We are hopeful that as further strides are made in understanding the psychobiology of OCD, so additional interventions will be developed, and the prognosis of this disorder further improved. In the interim, much can be done for patients with OCD using available technologies.

Chapter 7

Resources for patients and clinicians

7.1 Major rating scales for OCD

Y-BOCS   (see p. 87)
CY-BOCS   (see p. 101)
DY-BOCS   (see p. 117)
CGI   (see p. 147)

Zohar–Fineberg Obsessive Compulsive Screen (Z-FOCS): five screening questions for obsessive-compulsive disorder

1. Do you wash or clean a lot?
2. Do you check things a lot?
3. Is there any thought that keeps bothering you that you would like to get rid of but can't?
4. Do your daily activities take a long time to finish?
5. Are you concerned about orderliness or symmetry?

© Joseph Zohar and Naomi A. Fineberg, 2006.

7.2 Information and self-help books for children and adults with OCD, BDD and trichotillomania and their carers

Patients and their carers can benefit greatly from guided self-help using educational books and treatment manuals. There are a number of publications available. Below are just a few that the authors have found to be helpful.

7.2.1 OCD

7.2.1.1 Children

Wagner, P., Pinto, A. (2000). *Up and Down the Worry Hill: A Children's Book about Obsessive Compulsive Disorder and its Treatment.* Lighthouse Press, Lighthouse Point, Florida.

An illustrated book designed to help parents and professionals explain OCD to children through the story of 'Casey', a young boy with OCD.

Wever, C., Phillips, N. (1996). *The Secret Problem*.

A cartoon book that describes OCD in clear and simple language to help children, teenagers and parents understand OCD and its treatment.

7.2.1.2 *Adults and older adolescents*

Hyman, B., Pedrick, C. (2005). *The OCD Workbook: Your Guide to Breaking Free from Obsessive-Compulsive Disorder*. New Harbinger Publications, Oakland, CA.

A self-treatment manual for adults and older adolescents that guides the person with OCD through exposure with response prevention, with advice for family members.

Schwartz, J.M. (1997). *Brain Lock: Free Yourself from Obsessive Compulsive Behavior*. HarperCollins, New York.

A self-treatment manual suitable for adults and older adolescents with OCD.

Veale, D., Willson, R. (2005). *Overcoming Obsessive Compulsive Disorder*. Constable & Robinson, London.

A self-treatment book suitable for adults and older teenagers.

Tallis, F. (1992). *Understanding Obsessions and Compulsions: A Self-help Manual*. Sheldon Press, London.

A self-treatment book suitable for adults and older teenagers.

Rapaport, J. (1989). *The Boy who Couldn't Stop Washing: The Experience and Treatment of OCD*. Plume Books, New York.

Seminal text describing the experience and treatment of OCD.

7.2.2 **Body dysmorphic disorder**

Philips, K. (1996). *The Broken Mirror: Understanding and Treating Body Dysmorphic Disorder*. Oxford University Press, Oxford.

Describes the experience of BDD and discusses self-assessment, CBT and medication.

Claiborn, J., Pedrick, C. (2002). *The BDD Workbook: Overcome Body Dysmorphic Disorder and End Body Image Obsessions*. New Harbinger Publications, Oakland, CA.

A self-treatment book suitable for adults and older teenagers.

7.2.3 **Trichotillomania**

Keuthen, N., Stein, D., Christenson, G. (2001). Help for hairpullers: understanding and coping with trichotillomania. New Harbinger Publications, Oakland, CA.

A self-treatment book suitable for adults and older teenagers.

Penzel, F. (2003). *The Hair-pulling Problem; A Complete Guide to Trichotillomania*. Oxford University Press, Oxford.

Includes information on setting up a self-treatment programme with a section for parents.

7.2.4 Tourette's syndrome

Bruun, R. D., Bruun, B. (1994). *A Mind of Its Own: Tourette's Syndrome: A Story and a Guide*. Oxford University Press, Oxford.

Describes the experience of Tourette's. Suitable for adults and older teenagers.

7.2.5 Hypochondriasis

Cantor, C., Fallon, B. (1997). *Phantom Illness: Recognizing, Understanding, and Overcoming Hypochondria*. Houghton Mifflin, New York.

Autobiography, covering one woman's struggle with hypochondriasis and including many case examples and treatment strategies.

7.3 Information for healthcare practitioners

Clinicians may also benefit from reading the following:

7.3.1 OCD

Fineberg, N. Marazziti, D., Stein, D.J. eds (2001). *Obsessive Compulsive Disorder: A Practical Guide*. Martin Dunitz, London.

A practical guide for clinicians covering aetiology and treatment (CBT, medication and other forms of treatment).

Fineberg, N., Nigam, A. Obsessive-compulsive disorder: a guide to recognition and management. British Medical Journal online learning. http://www.bmjlearning.com/planrecord/servlet/ResourceSearch?key Word=obsessive&resourceId=5004330&viewResource=(accessed 27.11.06)

On-line resource for medical practitioners and allied professionals interested in learning more about recognition and clinical treatments for OCD.

Foa, E.F., March, J., Mulle, K. (1998). *OCD in Children and Adolescents: A Cognitive-Behavioural Treatment Manual*. Guilford Press, New York.

A manualized approach to CBT treatment of OCD including psycho-educational material and questionnaires.

Clark, D.A. *Cognitive Behavioural Therapy for OCD*. Guilford Press, New York.

Overview of cognitive and behavioural techniques for the treatment of OCD.

Heyman, I., Mataix-Cols, D., Fineberg, N.A. (2006 Aug 26). Obsessive-compulsive disorder. *Brit. Medical J.* **333**, 424–29.

Contemporary review for medical practitioners and allied professionals interested in neurobiological theories and clinical treatments for OCD.

7.3.2 **Body dysmorphic disorder**

Philips, K. (1996). *The Broken Mirror: Understanding and Treating Body Dysmorphic Disorder*. Oxford University Press, Oxford.

Describes the experience of BDD and discusses self-assessment, CBT approaches and medication.

7.3.3 **Trichotillomania**

Stein, D., Christenson, G., Hollander, E. (1999). *Trichotillomania*. American Psychiatric Publishing, Inc., Arlington, VA.

Describes the evaluation and treatment of compulsive hair-pulling.

7.4 Useful web sites for clinicians and patients

www.icocs.org
International College of Obsessive Compulsive Spectrum Disorders (ICOCS). Charity aimed at promoting collaborative research and raising the profile of OCD and OC-related disorders. Membership includes researchers, practitioners, individuals with OCD and their carers.

www.ocdyouth.info
Information on OCD and how to recover, for young people and their carers.

www.ocfoundation.org
OC Foundation: USA National Charity for OCD.

www.nice.org.uk
Web site for NICE Guidelines.

www.BAP.org
Web site for BAP Guidelines on Anxiety Disorders (including OCD).

7.5 Consumer associations involved in OCD

7.5.1 Australia

Anxiety Disorders Foundation of Australia, Inc.
www.senet.com.au/~adf/

Anxiety Recovery Centre Victoria
www.arcvic.com.au/index.html

Anxiety & Stress Management Service of Australia
www.anxietyhelp.com.au/

7.5.2 Canada

The Ontario Obsessive Compulsive Disorder Network (OOCDN)
www.oocdn.org

7.5.3 South Africa

Obsessive-Compulsive Disorder Association of South Africa.
P.O. Box 87127, Houghton, 2041, South Africa. Tel.: (+2711) 786–7030.
Fax, (12711) 706 5066.

7.5.4 **UK**

OCD Action
www.ocdaction.org.uk

OCD UK
www.ocduk.org/

First Steps to Freedom
www.first-steps.org/

7.5.5 **USA**

OC Foundation, Inc.
www.ocfoundation.org

Tourette Syndrome Association, Inc.
www.tsa-usa.org/

Appendix

Major rating scales for OCD

Yale–Brown Obsessive Compulsive Scale (Y-BOCS)

The Yale-Brown Obsessive Compulsive Scale (Y-BOCS) is a clinician-administered scale that assesses the type and severity of symptoms in patients with OCD. It is generally considered the best instrument currently available to clinicians for assessing treatment outcomes and symptom severity.

Y-BOCS is administered as a semi-structured interview and consists of a preliminary 64-item symptom checklist, followed by the main 19-item rating scale. The rating scale includes two main sub-scales – one measuring obsessions (items 1–5) and the other measuring compulsions (items 6–10) – which are used in determining the patient's total score. While the remaining items (11–19) are rated and may provide useful information to the clinician, they are not counted in the total score.

Reference

Goodman, W.K., Price, L.H., Rasmussen, S.A., et al. (1989). The Yale-Brown Obsessive Compulsive Scale. I. Development, use and reliability. *Archives of General Psychiatry* **46**: 1006–11.

Clinicians interested in using this scale and/or obtaining the full instructions should contact Dr Wayne K. Goodman, Department of Psychiatry, University of Florida College of Medicine, P.O. Box 100256, Gainesville, FL 32610, USA.

Name _____ Date _____

Y-BOCS SYMPTOM CHECKLIST (9/89)

Check all that apply, but clearly mark the principal symptoms with a 'P'.

(Rater must ascertain whether reported behaviours are bona-fide symptoms of OCD, and not symptoms of another disorder such as simple phobia or hypochondriasis. Items marked '*' may or may not be OCD phenomena.)

Current Past

AGGRESSIVE OBSESSIONS

____ ____ Fear might harm self

____ ____ Fear might harm others

____ ____ Violent or horrific images

____ ____ Fear of blurting out obscenities or insults

____ ____ Fear of doing something else embarrassing*

____ ____ Fear will act on unwanted impulses (e.g. to stab friend)

____ ____ Fear will steal things

____ ____ Fear will harm others because not careful enough (e.g. hit/run motor vehicle accident)

____ ____ Fear will be responsible for something else terrible happening (e.g. fire, burglary)

____ ____ Other _____

CONTAMINATION OBSESSIONS

____ ____ Concerns or disgust with bodily waste or secretions (e.g. urine, faeces, saliva)

____ ____ Concern with dirt or germs

____ ____ Excessive concern with environmental contaminants (e.g. asbestos, radiation, toxic waste)

____ ____ Excessive concern with household items (e.g. cleansers, solvents)

____ ____ Excessive concern with animals (e.g. insects)

____ ____ Bothered by sticky substances or residues

____ ____ Concerned will get ill because of contaminant

____ ____ Concerned will get others ill by spreading contaminant (aggressive)

____ ____ No concern with consequences of contamination other than how it might feel

____ ____ Other _____

SEXUAL OBSESSIONS
Forbidden or perverse sexual thoughts,
images, or impulses
____ ____ Content involves children or incest
____ ____ Content involves homosexuality*
____ ____ Sexual behaviour toward others (aggressive)*
____ ____ Other _____

HOARDING/SAVING OBSESSIONS
[distinguish from hobbies and concern with objects of monetary or
sentimental value]
____ ____ –

RELIGIOUS OBSESSIONS (Scrupulosity)
____ ____ Concerned with sacrilege and blasphemy
____ ____ Excess concern with right/wrong, morality
____ ____ Other _____

OBSESSION WITH NEED FOR SYMMETRY OR
EXACTNESS
Accompanied by magical thinking (e.g. concerned that
mother will have accident unless things are in the
____ ____ right place)
____ ____ Not accompanied by magical thinking

MISCELLANEOUS OBSESSIONS
____ ____ Need to know or remember
____ ____ Fear of saying certain things
____ ____ Fear of not saying just the right thing
____ ____ Fear of losing things
____ ____ Intrusive (non-violent) images
____ ____ Intrusive nonsense sounds, words, or music
____ ____ Bothered by certain sounds/noises*
____ ____ Lucky/unlucky numbers
____ ____ Colours with special significance
____ ____ Superstitious fears
____ ____ Other _____

SOMATIC OBSESSIONS
____ ____ Concern with illness or disease*
Excessive concern with body part or aspect of
____ ____ appearance (e.g. dysmorphophobia)*
____ ____ Other _____

Y–BOCS severity ratings

1. Time occupied by obsessive thoughts
0 = **None**.
1 = **Mild**, <1 hr/day or occasional intrusion.
2 = **Moderate**, 1 to 3 hr/day or frequent intrusion.
3 = **Severe**, >3 and up to 8 hr/day or very frequent intrusion.
4 = **Extreme**, >8 hr/day or near constant intrusion.

1b. Obsession-free interval (not included in total score)
0 = **No symptoms**.
1 = **Long symptom-free interval**, >8 consecutive hr/day symptom-free.
2 = **Moderately long symptom-free interval**, >3 and up to 8 consecutive hr/day symptom-free.
3 = **Short symptom-free interval**, from 1 to 3 consecutive hr/day symptom-free.
4 = **Extremely short symptom-free interval**, <1 consecutive hr/day symptom-free.

2. Interference due to obsessive thoughts
0 = **None**.
1 = **Mild**, slight interference with social or occupational activities, but overall performance not impaired.
2 = **Moderate**, definite interference with social or occupational performance, but still manageable.
3 = **Severe**, causes substantial impairment in social or occupational performance.
4 = **Extreme**, incapacitating.

3. Distress associated with obsessive thoughts
0 = **None**.
1 = **Mild**, not too disturbing.
2 = **Moderate**, disturbing, but still manageable.
3 = **Severe**, very disturbing.
4 = **Extreme**, near constant and disabling distress.

4. Resistance against obsessions
0 = **Makes an effort always to resist**, or symptoms so minimal doesn't need actively to resist.
1 = **Tries to resist most of the time**.
2 = **Makes some effort to resist**.
3 = **Yields to all obsessions** without attempting to control them, but does so with some reluctance.
4 = **Completely** and willingly yields to all obsessions.

92

Reproduced from Goodman, W.K., Price, L.H., Rasmussen, S.A., et al. (1989). Arch. Gen. Psych., **46**(11): 1006–11, with permission from the American Medical Association.

5. Degree of control over obsessive thoughts

0 = **Complete control.**

1 = **Much control,** usually able to stop or divert obsessions with some effort and concentration.

2 = **Moderate control,** sometimes able to stop or divert obsessions.

3 = **Little control,** rarely successful in stopping or dismissing obsessions, can only divert attention with difficulty.

4 = **No control,** experienced as completely involuntary, rarely able even momentarily to alter obsessive thinking.

6. Time spent performing compulsive behaviours

0 = **None.**

1 = **Mild** (spends <1 hr/day performing compulsions), or occasional performance of compulsive behaviours.

2 = **Moderate** (spends from 1 to 3 hr/day performing compulsions), or frequent performance of compulsive behaviours.

3 = **Severe** (spends >3 and up to 8 hr/day performing compulsions), or very frequent performance of compulsive behaviours.

4 = **Extreme** (spends >8 hr/day performing compulsions), or near constant performance of compulsive behaviours (too numerous to count).

6b. Compulsion-free interval (not included in total score)

0 = **No symptoms.**

1 = **Long symptom-free interval,** >8 consecutive hr/day symptom-free.

2 = **Moderately long symptom-free interval,** >3 and up to 8 consecutive hr/day symptom-free.

3 = **Short symptom-free interval,** from 1 to 3 consecutive hr/day symptom-free.

4 = **Extremely short symptom-free interval,** <1 consecutive hr/day symptom-free.

7. Interference due to compulsive behaviours

0 = **None.**

1 = **Mild,** slight interference with social or occupational activities, but overall performance not impaired.

2 = **Moderate,** definite interference with social or occupational performance, but still manageable.

3 = **Severe,** causes substantial impairment in social or occupational performance.

4 = **Extreme,** incapacitating.

8. *Distress associated with compulsive behaviour*

   0 = **None**.

   1 = **Mild** only slightly anxious if compulsions prevented, or only slight anxiety during performance of compulsions.

   2 = **Moderate**, reports that anxiety would mount but remain manageable if compulsions prevented, or that anxiety increases but remains manageable during performance of compulsions.

   3 = **Severe**, prominent and very disturbing increase in anxiety if compulsions interrupted, or prominent and very disturbing increase in anxiety during performance of compulsions.

   4 = **Extreme**, incapacitating anxiety from any intervention aimed at modifying activity, or incapacitating anxiety develops during performance of compulsions.

9. *Resistance against compulsions*

   0 = **Makes an effort to always resist**, or symptoms so minimal doesn't need actively to resist.

   1 = **Tries to resist most of the time**.

   2 = **Makes some effort to resist**.

   3 = **Yields to almost all compulsions** without attempting to control them, but does so with some reluctance.

   4 = **Completely and willingly yields** to all compulsions.

10. *Degree of control over compulsive behaviour*

    0 = **Complete control**.

    1 = **Much control**, experiences pressure to perform the behaviour but usually able to exercise voluntary control over it.

    2 = **Moderate control**, strong pressure to perform behaviour, can control it only with difficulty.

    3 = **Little control**, very strong drive to perform behaviour, must be carried to completion, can only delay with difficulty.

    4 = **No control**, drive to perform behaviour experienced as completely involuntary and overpowering, rarely able even momentarily to delay activity.

'The remaining questions are about both obsessions and compulsions. Some ask about related problems.' These are investigational items not included in total Y-BOCS score but may be useful in assessing these symptoms.

11. *Insight into obsessions and compulsions*

    0 = **Excellent insight**, fully rational.

    1 = **Good insight**. Readily acknowledges absurdity or excessiveness of thoughts or behaviours but does not seem

completely convinced that there isn't something besides
anxiety to be concerned about (i.e. has lingering doubts).

2 = **Fair insight**. Reluctantly admits thoughts or behaviour
seem unreasonable or excessive, but wavers. May have
some unrealistic fears, but no fixed convictions.

3 = **Poor insight**. Maintains that thoughts or behaviours are
not unreasonable or excessive, but acknowledges validity
of contrary evidence (i.e. overvalued ideas present).

4 = **Lacks insight**, delusional. Definitely convinced that
concerns and behaviour are reasonable, unresponsive to
contrary evidence.

2. *Avoidance*

0 = **No** deliberate avoidance.

1 = **Mild**, minimal avoidance.

2 = **Moderate**, some avoidance; clearly present.

3 = **Severe**, much avoidance; avoidance prominent.

4 = **Extreme**, very extensive avoidance; patient does almost
everything he/she can to avoid triggering symptoms.

3. *Degree of indecisiveness*

0 = **None**.

1 = **Mild**, some trouble in making decisions about minor things.

2 = **Moderate**, freely reports significant trouble in making
decisions that others would not think twice about.

3 = **Severe**, continual weighing of pros and cons about
non-essentials.

4 = **Extreme**, unable to make any decisions. Disabling.

4. *Overvalued sense of responsibility*

0 = **None**.

1 = **Mild**, only mentioned on questioning, slight sense of
over-responsibility.

2 = **Moderate**, ideas stated spontaneously, clearly present;
patient experiences significant sense of over-responsibility
for events outside his/her reasonable control.

3 = **Severe**, ideas prominent and pervasive; deeply concerned
he/she is responsible for events clearly outside his
control. Self-blaming farfetched and nearly irrational.

4 = **Extreme**, delusional sense of responsibility (e.g. if an
earthquake occurs 3000 miles away patient blames herself
because she didn't perform her compulsions).

5. *Pervasive slowness/ disturbance of inertia*

0 = **None**.

1 = **Mild**, occasional delay in starting or finishing.

2 = **Moderate**, frequent prolongation of routine activities but tasks usually completed. Frequently late.

3 = **Severe**, pervasive and marked difficulty initiating and completing routine tasks. Usually late.

4 = **Extreme**, unable to start or complete routine tasks without full assistance.

16. *Pathological doubting*

0 = **None**.

1 = **Mild**, only mentioned on questioning, slight pathological doubt. Examples given may be within normal range.

2 = **Moderate**, ideas stated spontaneously, clearly present and apparent in some of patient's behaviours; patient bothered by significant pathological doubt. Some effect on performance but still manageable.

3 = **Severe**, uncertainty about perceptions or memory rominent; pathological doubt frequently affects performance.

4 = **Extreme**, uncertainty about perceptions constantly present; pathological doubt substantially affects almost all activities. Incapacitating (e.g. patient states 'my mind doesn't trust what my eyes see').

[Items 17 and 18 refer to global illness severity. The rater is require to consider global function, not just the severity of obsessive compulsive symptoms.]

17. *Global severity:* Interviewer's judgement of the overall severity c the patient's illness.

0 = **No illness**.

1 = **Illness slight**, doubtful, transient; no functional impairment.

2 = **Mild symptoms**, little functional impairment.

3 = **Moderate symptoms**, functions with effort.

4 = **Moderate – severe symptoms**, limited functioning.

5 = **Severe symptoms**, functions mainly with assistance.

6 = **Extremely severe symptoms**, completely non-functional.

18. *Global improvement:* Interviewer's judgement of the total overal improvement present since the initial rating whether or not, i your judgement, it is due to drug treatment.

0 = **Very much worse**.

1 = **Much worse**.

2 = **Minimally worse**.

3 = **No change**.

4 = **Minimally improved**.

5 = **Much improved**.

6 = **Very much improved**.

19. *Reliability:* Interviewer's judgement of the overall reliability of the rating scores obtained.

0 = **Excellent**, no reason to suspect data unreliable.
1 = **Good**, factor(s) present that may adversely affect reliability.
2 = **Fair**, factor(s) present that definitely reduce reliability.
3 = **Poor**, very low reliability.

Items 17 and 18 are adapted from the Clinical Global Impression Scale (Guy, W. (1976) *ECDEU Assessment Manual for Psychopharmacology: Publication 76–338*. US Department of Health, Education, and Welfare, Washington, D.C.)

Yale-Brown Obsessive Compulsive Scale (9/89)
Y-BOCS TOTAL (add items 1–10)

Patient name _____   Date _____

Patient ID _____   Rater _____

		None	Mild	Moderate	Severe	Extreme
1.	Time spent on obsessions	0	1	2	3	4

1b. Obsession-free interval

		No symptoms	Long	Moderately long	Short	Extremely short
	(do not add to subtotal or total score)	0	1	2	3	4

		None	Mild	Moderate	Severe	Extreme
2.	Interference from obsessions	0	1	2	3	4
3.	Distress of obsessions	0	1	2	3	4

		Always Resists				Completely yields
4.	Resistance	0	1	2	3	4

		Complete control	Much control	Moderate control	Little control	No control
5.	Control over obsessions	0	1	2	3	4

OBSESSION SUBTOTAL (add items 1–5)

		None	Mild	Moderate	Severe	Extreme
6.	Time spent on compulsions	0	1	2	3	4

6b. Compulsion-free interval

		No Symptoms	Long	Moderately long	Short	Extremely short
	(do not add to subtotal or total score)	0	1	2	3	4

		None	Mild	Moderate	Severe	Extreme
7.	Interference from compulsions	0	1	2	3	4
8.	Distress from compulsions	0	1	2	3	4

		Always Resists		Completely yields		
9.	Resistance	0	1	2	3	4

		Complete control	Much control	Moderate control	Little control	No control
10.	Control over compulsions	0	1	2	3	4

COMPULSION SUBTOTAL (add items 6–10)

Reproduced from Goodman, W.K., Price, L.H., Rasmussen, S.A., et al. (1989). *Arch. Gen. Psych.*, **46**(11): 1006–11, with permission from the American Medical Association.

		Excellent				Absent
11.	Insight into O-C symptoms	0	1	2	3	4

		None	Mild	Moderate	Severe	Extreme
12.	Avoidance	0	1	2	3	4
13.	Indecisiveness	0	1	2	3	4
14.	Pathological responsibility	0	1	2	3	4
15.	Slowness	0	1	2	3	4
16.	Pathological doubting	0	1	2	3	4

17.	Global severity	0	1	2	3	4	5	6
18.	Global improvement	0	1	2	3	4	5	6

19. Reliability   Excellent = 0   Good = 1   Fair = 2   Poor = 3

APPENDIX Major rating scales for OCD

Children's Yale–Brown Obsessive Compulsive Scale (CY-BOCS)

The Children's Yale Brown Obsessive Compulsive Scale (CY-BOCS) is a commonly used clinician-rated scale of paediatric obsessive compulsive symptom severity. It is a modified version of the original Y-BOCS scale.

Reference
Goodman WK, Price LH, Rasmussen SA, *et al.* (1989) The Yale-Brown Obsessive Compulsive Scale. I. Development, use and reliability. *Arch. Gen. Psych.* **46**: 1006–11.

CY-BOCS Obsessions Checklist

(1)	X	Contamination obsessions	Current	Past	Trauma-related	Non-trauma-related
		Concern with dirt, germs, certain illnesses (e.g. AIDS)				
		Concern or disgust with bodily waste or secretions (e.g. urine, faeces, saliva)				
		Excessive concern with environmental contaminants (e.g. asbestos, radiation, toxic waste)				
		Excessive concern with household items (e.g. cleaners, solvents)				
		Excessively bothered by sticky substances or residues				
		Concerned will get ill because of contaminant				
		Concerned will get others ill by spreading contaminant				
		No concern with consequences of contamination other than how it might feel*				

(2)	X	Aggressive obsessions	Current	Past	Trauma-related	Non-trauma-related
		Fear might harm self				
		Fear might harm others				
		Fear harm will come to self				
		Fear harm will come to others (may be because of something child did or did not do)				
		Violent or horrific images				
		Fear of blurting out obscenities or insults				
		Fear of doing something else embarrassing*				
		Fear will act on unwanted impulses (e.g. to stab a family member)				
		Fear will steal things				

102

Reproduced with permission from Dr Wayne J. Goodman.

Fear will be responsible for something else terrible happening (e.g. fire, burglary, flood)

3) X	Sexual obsessions	Current	Past	Trauma-related	Non-trauma-related

Ask the child, 'Are you having any sexual thoughts?' If yes,

'Are they routine or are they repetitive thoughts that you would rather not have or find disturbing?' If yes,

'Are they ...'Forbidden or perverse sexual thoughts, images, or impulses

Content involves homosexuality

Sexual behaviour towards others (aggressive)

4) X	Hoarding/saving obsessions	Current	Past	Trauma-related	Non-trauma-related

Fear of losing things

5) X	Magical thoughts/superstitious obsessions	Current	Past	Trauma-related	Non-trauma-related

Lucky/unlucky numbers, colours, words

6) X	Somatic obsessions	Current	Past	Trauma-related	Non-trauma-related

Excessive concern with illness or disease*

Excessive concern with body part or aspect of appearance (e.g. dysmorphophobia)

7) X	Religious obsessions	Current	Past	Trauma-related	Non-trauma-related

Excessive concern or fear of offending religious objects (God)

Excessive concern with
right/wrong, morality

(8)	X	Miscellaneous obsessions	Current	Past	Trauma-related	Non-trauma-related

The need to know or
remember

Fear of saying certain things

Fear of not saying just the
right thing

Intrusive (non-violent) images

Intrusive sounds, words,
music or numbers

Target symptom list for obsessions

Please list the obsessions experienced. Note if absent.	Trauma-related	Non-trauma-related

1.

2.

3.

4.

CY-BOCS Compulsions Checklist

Check all symptoms that apply.

Washing/cleaning compulsions	Current	Past	TR	NTR
Excessive or ritualized hand washing				
Excessive or ritualized showering, bathing, tooth brushing, grooming, toilet routine				
Excessive cleaning of items (such as personal clothes or important objects)				
Other measures to prevent or remove contact with contaminants				
Other (describe)				

Checking compulsions	Current	Past	TR	NTR
Checking locks, toys, school books/items, etc				
Checking associated with getting washed, dressed, or undressed				
Checking that did not/will not harm others				
Checking that did not/will not harm self				
Checking that nothing terrible did/will happen				
Checking that did not make a mistake				
Checking tied to somatic obsessions				
Other				

Repeating rituals	Current	Past	TR	NTR
Rereading, erasing, or rewriting				
Need to repeat routine activities (e.g. in/out of doorway, up/down from chair)				
Other				

Counting compulsions	Current	Past	TR	NTR
Objects, certain numbers, words, etc.				
Other				

Ordering/arranging	Current	Past	TR	NTR
Need for symmetry/evening up (e.g. lining items up a certain way or arranging personal items in specific patterns)				
Other				

105

Hoarding/saving compulsions	Current	Past	TR	NTR
Distinguish from hobbies and concern with objects of monetary or sentimental value				
Difficulty throwing things away, saving bits of paper, string, etc.				
Other				

Excessive games/superstitious behaviours	Current	Past	TR	NTR
Distinguish from age-appropriate magical games (e.g. array of behaviour, such as stepping over certain spots on a floor, touching an object/self certain number of times as a routine game to avoid something bad from happening)				
Other				

Rituals involving other persons	Current	Past	TR	NTR
The need to involve another person (usually a parent) in ritual (e.g. asking a parent to repeatedly answer the same question, making mother perform certain meal time rituals involving specific utensils)				
Other (describe)				

Miscellaneous compulsions	Current	Past	TR	NTR
Mental rituals (other than checking/counting)				
The need to tell, ask, or confess				
Measures (not checking) to prevent harm to self, harm to others, or terrible consequences				
Ritualized eating behaviours*				
Excessive list making*				
Need to touch, tap, rub*				
Need to do things (e.g. touch or arrange) until it feels just right*				
Rituals involving blinking or staring*				
Trichotillomania (hair-pulling)*				
Other self-damaging or self-mutilating behaviours				
Other				

Target symptom list for compulsions

Please list the compulsions experienced. Note if absent.	TR	NTR
1.		
2.		
3.		
4.		

Source: Children's Yale–Brown Obsessive Compulsive Scale, W.K. Goodman et al., second revision, 5/1/1991.

1. Are the obsessions part of the principal/target symptoms? [Yes | No]

2. Are the compulsions part of the principal/target symptoms? [Yes | No]

3. When did the trauma related obsessions begin?

4. When did the non-trauma-related obsessions begin?

5. When did the trauma-related compulsions begin?

6. When did the non-trauma-related compulsions begin?

CY-BOCS severity ratings

1. Time occupied by obsessive thoughts

0 = **None**.
1 = **Mild**, <1 hr/day or occasional intrusion.
2 = **Moderate**, 1–3 hr/day or frequent intrusion.
3 = **Severe**, >3 and up to 8 hr/day or very frequent intrusion.
4 = **Extreme**, >8 hr/day or near constant intrusion.

1B. Obsession-free interval (not included in total score)

0 = **None**.
1 = **Mild**, Long symptom-free intervals, >8 consecutive hr/day symptom-free.
2 = **Moderate**, Moderately long symptom-free intervals, >3 and up to 8 consecutive hr/day symptom-free.
3 = **Severe**, Brief symptom-free intervals, from 1 to 3 consecutive hr/day symptom-free.
4 = **Extreme**, <1 consecutive hr/day symptom-free.

2. Interference due to obsessive thoughts

0 = **None**.
1 = **Mild**, Slight interference with social or school activities, but overall performance not impaired.
2 = **Moderate**, definite interference with social or school performance, but still manageable.
3 = **Severe**, causes substantial impairment in social or school performance.
4 = **Extreme**, incapacitating.

3. Distress associated with obsessive thoughts

0 = **None**
1 = **Mild**, infrequent, and not too disturbing.
2 = **Moderate**, frequent, and disturbing, but still manageable.
3 = **Severe**, very frequent, and very disturbing.
4 = **Extreme**, near constant, and disabling distress/frustration.

4. Resistance against obsessions

0 = **None**, makes an effort always to resist, or symptoms so minimal doesn't need to actively resist.
1 = **Mild**, tries to resist most of the time.
2 = **Moderate**, makes some effort to resist.
3 = **Severe**, yields to all obsessions without attempting to control them, but does so with some reluctance.
4 = **Extreme**, completely and willingly yields to all obsessions.

Reproduced with permission from Dr Wayne J. Goodman.

5. *Degree of control over obsessive thoughts*
0 = **Complete control**.
1 = **Much control**, usually able to stop or divert obsessions with some effort and concentration.
2 = **Moderate control**, sometimes able to stop or divert obsessions.
3 = **Little control**, rarely successful in stopping obsessions, can only divert attention with difficulty.
4 = **No control**, experienced as completely involuntary, rarely able even momentarily to divert thinking.

Questions on Compulsions (Items 6–10)

6A. *Time spent performing compulsive behaviours*
0 = **None**.
1 = **Mild**, spends less than 1 hr/day performing compulsions, or occasional performance of compulsive behaviours.
2 = **Moderate**, spends from 1 to 3 hr/day performing compulsions, or frequent performance of compulsions.
3 = **Severe**, spends more than 3 and up to 8 hr/day performing compulsions, or very frequent performance of compulsions.
4 = **Extreme**, spends >8 hr/day performing compulsions, or near constant performance of compulsive behaviours (to numerous to count).

6B. Compulsion-free interval

0 = **No symptoms**.

1 = **Mild**, long symptom-free interval, >8 consecutive hr/day symptom-free.

2 = **Moderate**, moderately long symptom-free interval, >3 and up to 8 consecutive hr/day symptom-free.

3 = **Severe**, short symptom-free interval, from 1 to 3 consecutive hr/day symptom-free.

4 = **Extreme**, <1 consecutive hr/day symptom-free.

7. Interference due to compulsive behaviours

0 = **None**.

1 = **Mild**, slight interference with social or school activities, but overall performance not impaired.

2 = **Moderate**, definite interference with social or school performance, but still manageable.

3 = **Severe**, causes substantial impairment in social or school performance.

4 = **Extreme**, incapacitating.

8. Distress associated with compulsive behaviour

0 = **None**.

1 = **Mild**, only slightly anxious/frustrated if compulsions prevented, or only slight anxiety/frustration during performance of compulsions.

2 = **Moderate**, reports that anxiety/frustration would mount but remain manageable if compulsions prevented. Anxiety/frustration increases but remains manageable during performance of compulsions.

3 = **Severe**, prominent and very disturbing increase in anxiety/frustration if compulsions interrupted. Prominent and very disturbing increase in anxiety/frustration during performance of compulsions.

4 = **Extreme**, Incapacitating anxiety/frustration from any intervention aimed at modifying activity. Incapacitating anxiety/frustration develops during performance of compulsions.

9. Resistance against compulsions

0 = **None**, makes an effort always to resist, or symptoms so minimal doesn't need to actively resist.

1 = **Mild**, tries to resist most of the time.

2 = **Moderate**, makes some effort to resist.

3 = **Severe**, yields to almost all compulsions without attempting to control them, but does so with some reluctance.

4 = **Extreme**, completely and willingly yields to all compulsions.

10. *Degree of control over compulsive behaviour*

    0 = **Complete control.**

    1 = **Much control,** experiences pressure to perform the behaviour, but usually able to exercise voluntary control over it.

    2 = **Moderate control,** moderate control, strong pressure to perform behaviour, can control it only with difficulty.

    3 = **Little control,** little control, very strong drive to perform behaviour, must be carried to completion, can only delay with difficulty.

    4 = **No control,** no control, drive to perform behaviour experienced as completely involuntary and overpowering, rarely able to delay activity (even momentarily).

11. *Insight into obsessions and compulsions*

    0 = **None,** excellent insight, fully rational.

    1 = **Mild,** good insight, readily acknowledges absurdity or excessiveness of thoughts or behaviours but does not seem completely convinced that there isn't something besides anxiety to be concerned about (i.e. has lingering doubts).

    2 = **Moderate,** fair insight, reluctantly admits thoughts or behaviour seem unreasonable or excessive, but wavers. May have some unrealistic fears, but no fixed convictions.

    3 = **Severe,** poor insight, maintains that thoughts or behaviours are not reasonable or excessive, but wavers. May have some unrealistic fears, but acknowledges validity of contrary evidence (i.e. overvalued ideas present).

    4 = **Extreme,** lacks insight, delusional, definitely convinced that concerns and behaviour are reasonable, unresponsive to contrary evidence.

12. *Avoidance*

    0 = **None.**

    1 = **Mild,** minimal avoidance.

    2 = **Moderate,** some avoidance; clearly present.

    3 = **Severe,** much avoidance; avoidance prominent.

    4 = **Extreme,** very extensive avoidance; patient does almost everything he/she can to avoid triggering symptoms.

13. *Degree of indecisiveness*

    0 = **None.**

    1 = **Mild,** some trouble making decisions about minor things.

    2 = **Moderate,** freely reports significant trouble in making decisions that others would not think twice about.

    3 = **Severe,** continual weighing of pros and cons about non- essentials.

    4 = **Extreme,** unable to make any decisions, disabling.

14. Overvalued sense of responsibility
0 = **None**.

1 = **Mild**, Only mentioned on questioning, slight sense of over-responsibility.

2 = **Moderate**, Ideas stated spontaneously, clearly present; patient experiences significant sense of over-responsibility for events outside his/her reasonable control.

3 = **Severe**, Ideas prominent and pervasive; deeply concerned he/she is responsible for events clearly outside his control, self-blaming farfetched and nearly irrational.

4 = **Extreme**, Delusional sense of responsibility (e.g. if an earthquake occurs 3000 miles away patient blames himself because he didn't perform his compulsion).

15. Pervasive slowness/disturbance of Inertia
0 = **None**.

1 = **Mild**, occasional delay in starting or finishing tasks/activities.

2 = **Moderate**, frequent prolongation of routine activities but tasks usually completed, frequently late.

3 = **Severe**, pervasive and marked difficulty initiating and completing routine tasks, usually late.

4 = **Extreme**, unable to start or complete routine tasks without full assistance.

16. Pathological doubting
0 = **None**.

1 = **Mild**, only mentioned on questioning, slight pathological doubt, examples given may be within normal range.

2 = **Moderate**, ideas stated spontaneously, clearly present and apparent in some of patient's behaviours; patient bothered by significant pathological doubt. Some effect on performance but still manageable.

3 = **Severe**, uncertainty about perceptions or memory prominent; pathological doubt frequently affects performance.

4 = **Extreme**, uncertainty about perceptions constantly present; pathological doubt substantially affects almost all activities, incapacitating (e.g. patient states "my mind doesn't trust what my eyes see").

17. Global severity
Interviewer's judgement of the overall severity of the patient's illness. Rated from 0 (no illness) to 6 (most severe patient seen). (Consider the degree of distress reported by the patient, the symptoms observed and the functional impairment reported. Your judgement is required both in averaging these data as well as weighing the reliability or accuracy of the data obtained.)

0 = **No illness.**
1 = **Slight**, illness slight, doubtful, transient; no functional impairment.
2 = **Mild**, little functional impairment.
3 = **Moderate**, functions with effort.
4 = **Moderate–severe**, limited functioning.
5 = **Severe**, functions mainly with assistance
6 = **Extremely severe**, completely non-functional.

18. Global improvement

Rate total overall improvement present since the initial rating whether or not, in your judgement, it is due to treatment.

0 = **Very much worse.**
1 = **Much worse.**
2 = **Minimally worse.**
3 = **No change.**
4 = **Minimally improved.**
5 = **Much improved.**
6 = **Very much improved.**

19. Reliability

Rate the overall reliability of the rating scores obtained. Factors that may affect reliability include the patient's cooperativeness and his/her natural ability to communicate. The type and severity of obsessive-compulsive symptoms present may interfere with the patient's concentration, attention, or freedom to speak spontaneously (e.g. the content of some obsessions may cause the patient to choose his words very carefully).

0 = **Excellent**, no reason to suspect data unreliable.
1 = **Good**, factor(s) present that may adversely affect reliability.
2 = **Fair**, factor(s) present that definitely reduce reliability.
3 = **Poor**, very low reliability.

Children's Yale–Brown Obsessive Compulsive Scale
CY-BOCS TOTAL (add items 1–10)

Patient name _____ Date _____

Patient ID _____ Rater _____

	None	Mild	Moderate	Severe	Extreme
1. Time spent on obsessions	0	1	2	3	4

	No symptoms	Long	Moderately long	Short	Extremely short
1b. Obsession-free interval (do not add to subtotal or total score)	0	1	2	3	4

	None	Mild	Moderate	Severe	Extreme
2. Interference from obsessions	0	1	2	3	4
3. Distress of obsessions	0	1	2	3	4

	Always Resists				Completely yields
4. Resistance	0	1	2	3	4

	Complete control	Much control	Moderate control	Little control	No control
5. Control over obsessions	0	1	2	3	4

OBSESSION SUBTOTAL (add items 1–5) | TR | NTR |

	None	Mild	Moderate	Severe	Extreme
6. Time spent on compulsions	0	1	2	3	4

	No Symptoms	Long	Moderately long	Short	Extremely short
6b. Compulsion-free interval (do not add to sub-total or total score)	0	1	2	3	4

	None	Mild	Moderate	Severe	Extreme
7. Interference from compulsions	0	1	2	3	4

8. Distress from compulsions	0	1	2	3	4	

	Always Resists				Completely yields

9. Resistance	0	1	2	3	4

	Complete control	Much control	Moderate control	Little control	No control
10. Control over compulsions	0	1	2	3	4

COMPULSION SUBTOTAL (add items 6–10) | TR | NTR

	Excellent				Absent
11. Insight into O-C symptoms	0	1	2	3	4

	None	Mild	Moderate	Severe	Extreme
12. Avoidance	0	1	2	3	4
13. Indecisiveness	0	1	2	3	4
14. Pathological responsibility	0	1	2	3	4
15. Slowness	0	1	2	3	4
16. Pathological doubting	0	1	2	3	4

17. Global severity	0	1	2	3	4	5	6
18. Global improvement	0	1	2	3	4	5	6

19. Reliability   Excellent = 0   Good = 1   Fair = 2   Poor = 3

Dimensional Yale–Brown Obsessive Compulsive Severity Scale (DY-BOCS)

The Dimensional Yale-Brown Obsessive Compulsive Scale (DY-BOCS) is an extension of the original Yale-Brown Obsessive Compulsive Scale (Y-BOCS) that is designed to evaluate the nature and current severity of obsessive-compulsive symptoms. DY-BOCS inclu des specific symptom checklists/severity ratings for the following symptom categories: 1) aggressive obsessions and related compulsions; 2) sexual and religious obsessions and related compulsions; 3) symmetry, ordering, counting, and arranging obsessions and compulsions; 4) contamination obsessions and cleaning compulsions; 5) hoarding and collecting obsessions and compulsions; 6) somatic obsessions and compulsions; and 7) miscellaneous symptoms.

References

Goodman, W.K., Price, L.H., Rasmussen, S.A., et al. (1989). The Yale-Brown Obsessive Compulsive Scale. I. Development, use and reliability. *Archives in General Psychiatry* **46**: 1006–11.

Leckman, J.F., Grice, D.E., Boardman, J., et al. (1997). Symptoms of obsessive-compulsive disorder. *American Journal of Psychiatry* **154**(7): 911–7.

Mataix-Cols, D., Rauch, S.L., Manzo, P.A., et al. (1999). Use of factor-analyzed symptom dimensions to predict outcome with serotonin reuptake inhibitors and placebo in the treatment of obsessive-compulsive disorder. *American Journal of Psychiatry* **156**(9): 1409–16.

Summerfeldt, L.J., Richter, M.A., Antony, M.M., Swinson, R.P. (1999). Symptom structure in obsessive-compulsive disorder: a confirmatory factor-analytic study. *Behav. Res. Ther.* **37**(4): 297–311.

Severity ratings (past week) for aggressive obsessions and related compulsions

1. *How much of your time is occupied by these obsessions and compulsions?*
   - 0 = **No time at all.**
   - 1 = **Rarely**, present during the past week, often not on a daily basis, typically <3 hr/week.
   - 2 = **Occasionally, >3 hr/week, but <1 hr/day** – occasional intrusion, need to perform compulsions, or avoidance (occurs no >5 times a day).
   - 3 = **Frequently, 1 to 3 hr/day** – frequent intrusion, need to perform compulsions, or avoidance (occurs >8 times a day, but most hours of the day are free of these obsessions, compulsions, and related avoidance).
   - 4 = **Almost always, >3 and up to 8 hr/day** – very frequent intrusion, need to perform compulsions, or avoidance (occurs >8 times a day and occurs during most hours of the day).
   - 5 = **Always, >8 hr/day** – near constant intrusion of obsessions, need to perform compulsions, or avoidance (too numerous to count and an hour rarely passes without several obsessions, compulsions and/or avoidance).

2. *How much distress do these obsessions and related compulsions cause?*
   - 0 = **No distress**.
   - 1 = **Minimal**, when symptoms are present they are minimally distressing.
   - 2 = **Mild**, some clear distress present, but not too disturbing.
   - 3 = **Moderate**, disturbing, but still tolerable.
   - 4 = **Severe**, very disturbing.
   - 5 = **Extreme**, near constant and disabling distress.

3. *How much do these obsessions and related compulsions interfere with your family life, friendships, or ability to perform well at work or at school?*
   - 0 = **No interference.**
   - 1 = **Minimal**, slight interference with social or occupational activities, overall performance not impaired.
   - 2 = **Mild**, some interference with social or occupational activities, overall performance affected to a small degree.
   - 3 = **Moderate**, definite interference with social or occupational performance but still manageable.
   - 4 = **Severe interference**, causes substantial impairment in social or occupational performance.
   - 5 = **Extreme**, incapacitating interference.

Reproduced with permission from Dr James Leckman.

Checklist of sexual and religious obsessions and related compulsions severity ratings (past week)

Checklist check once (✓) for any symptoms present during the past week.

Here the emphasis is on obsessions and compulsions based on sexual and religious concerns. Moral concerns that are not explicitly religious in character belong in this category as well. There may be some inherent overlap with the aggressive domain. However, check items in this category if the primary issue concerns sexual, moral or religious matters.

Obsessions with sexual content
___ Forbidden or improper sexual thoughts
___ Content involves children or incest
___ Content involves homosexuality

___ Content involves violent sexual acts

Related compulsions
___ Checking compulsions related to sexual obsessions

___ Repeating compulsions related to sexual obsessions
___ Mental rituals related to sexual obsessions

Avoidance because of sexual obsessions
___ Intentional avoidance of people, places or things because of any of the above obsessions or compulsions concerning sex

Obsessions with religious content*
___ Content involves sacrilege or blasphemy

___ Excessive concern with what is morally right or wrong
___ Fear saying certain things
___ Need to tell, ask or confess things

Related compulsions
___ Checking or other compulsions related to religious obsessions

___

___ Repeating compulsions related to religious obsessions
___ Mental rituals related to religious obsessions

Avoidance – religious
___ Intentional avoidance of people, places or things because of any of the above obsessions or compulsions concerning religious topics

Other obsessions or compulsions in this category (describe):

_____

_____

Symptoms in this category were present during the past week?
   Yes   No
If yes, complete the next page. If no, skip to next section.

Severity ratings (past week) for sexual and religious obsessions and related compulsions

1. *How much of your time is occupied by these obsessions and compulsions?*
   - 0 = **No time at all.**
   - 1 = **Rarely** present during the past week, often not on a daily basis, typically <3 hr/week.
   - 2 = **Occasionally, >3 hr/week, but <1 hr/day** – occasional intrusion, need to perform compulsions, or avoidance (occurs no >5 times a day).
   - 3 = **Frequently, 1 to 3 hr/day** – frequent intrusion, need to perform compulsions, or avoidance (occurs >8 times a day, but most hours of the day are free of these obsessions, compulsions, and related avoidance).
   - 4 = **Almost always, >3 and up to 8 hr/day** – very frequent intrusion, need to perform compulsions, or avoidance (occurs >8 times a day and occurs during most hours of the day).
   - 5 = **Always, >8 hr/day** – near constant intrusion of obsessions, need to perform compulsions, or avoidance (too numerous to count and an hour rarely passes without several obsessions, compulsions and/or avoidance).

2. *How much distress do these obsessions and related compulsions cause?*
   - 0 = **No distress.**
   - 1 = **Minimal,** when symptoms are present they are minimally distressing.
   - 2 = **Mild,** some clear distress present, but not too disturbing.
   - 3 = **Moderate,** disturbing, but still tolerable.
   - 4 = **Severe,** very disturbing.
   - 5 = **Extreme,** near constant and disabling distress.

3. *How much do these obsessions and related compulsions interfere with your family life, friendships, or ability to perform well at work or at school?*

0 = **No interference**.

1 = **Minimal**, slight interference with social or occupational activities, overall performance not impaired.

2 = **Mild**, some interference with social or occupational activities, overall performance affected to a small degree.

3 = **Moderate**, definite interference with social or occupational performance but still manageable.

4 = **Severe interference**, causes substantial impairment in social or occupational performance.

5 = **Extreme**, incapacitating interference.

Checklist of symmetry, ordering, counting, and arranging obsessions and compulsions (past week)

Checklist check once (✓) for any symptoms present during the past week.

This dimension is usually fairly distinctive when present. However, overlaps can occur with other dimensions, particularly when there are concerns about harm or illness. Check these items only if in your best judgement the symptoms are best accounted for under this category. Similarly, if you are uncertain about which category best covers the symptoms in question, please indicate your doubts with annotations and rate the symptoms accordingly in more than one dimension.

Obsessions
___ Content involves needing things to be perfect or exact or 'just right'
___ Content involves needing things to be symmetrical or correctly aligned
___ Fear not saying 'just the right thing'

Compulsions
___ Checking for own mistakes

___ Ordering and arranging compulsions

___ Compulsions involving touching, tapping or rubbing
___ Compulsions involving evening-up, or aligning Re-reading or rewriting compulsions
___ Repeating routine activities
___ Counting compulsions
___ Other mental rituals

Avoidance
___ Intentional avoidance of places or things because of these obsessions or compulsions
Other symptoms in this category (describe):

_____

_____

_____

Symptoms in this category were present during the past week?
    Yes   No
If yes, complete the next page. If no, skip to next section.

Severity (past week) of symmetry, ordering, counting, and arranging obsessions and compulsions

1. *How much of your time is occupied by these obsessions and compulsions?*
   - 0 = **No time at all**.
   - 1 = **Rarely** present during the past week, often not on a daily basis, typically <3 hr/week.
   - 2 = **Occassionally, >3 hr/week, but <1 hr/day** – occasional intrusion, need to perform compulsions, or avoidance (occurs no >5 times a day).
   - 3 = **Frequently, 1 to 3 hr/day** – frequent intrusion, need to perform compulsions, or avoidance (occurs >8 times a day, but most hours of the day are free of these obsessions, compulsions, and related avoidance).
   - 4 = **Almost always, >3 and up to 8 hr/day** – very frequent intrusion, need to perform compulsions, or avoidance (occurs >8 times a day and occurs during most hours of the day).
   - 5 = **Always, >8 hr/day** – near constant intrusion of obsessions, need to perform compulsions, or avoidance (too numerous to count and an hour rarely passes without several obsessions, compulsions and/or avoidance).

2. *How much distress do these obsessions and related compulsions cause you?*
   - 0 = **No distress**.
   - 1 = **Minimal**, when symptoms are present they are minimally distressing.
   - 2 = **Mild**, some clear distress present, but not too disturbing.
   - 3 = **Moderate**, disturbing but still tolerable.
   - 4 = **Severe**, very disturbing.
   - 5 = **Extreme**, near constant and disabling distress.

3. *How much do these obsessions and related compulsions interfere with your family life, friendships, or ability to perform well at work or at school?*

   0 = **No interference**.

   1 = **Minimal**, slight interference with social or occupational activities, overall performance not impaired.

   2 = **Mild**, some interference with social or occupational activities, overall performance affected to a small degree.

   3 = **Moderate**, definite interference with social or occupational performance but still manageable.

   4 = **Severe interference**, causes substantial impairment in social or occupational performance.

   5 = **Extreme**, incapacitating interference.

Checklist of contamination obsessions and cleaning compulsions

Checklist check once (✓) for any symptoms present during the past week.

Again, this category is usually quite distinctive when present and in some individuals it is the only dimension present. Care may be needed to distinguish between aggressive and somatic obsessions. Check only if clear obsessions or compulsions that include contamination content are present.

Obsessions

___ Content involves dirt and germs

___ Concerns or disgust with bodily waste or secretions

___ Content involves environmental household contaminants

___ Content involves insects or animals

___ Bothered by sticky substances

___ Content involves worry about becoming ill because of contamination

Compulsions

___ Compulsive or ritualized hand washing

___ Repeated cleaning of household items or other inanimate objects

___ Ritualized showering, bathing, or toilet routines

___ Measures taken to prevent contact with household contaminants

___ Mental rituals associated with contamination

Avoidance

___ Intentional avoidance of places or things because of these obsessions or compulsions

Other symptoms in this category (describe):

_____

_____

Symptoms in this category were present during the past week?
   Yes   No
If yes, complete the next page. If no, skip to next section.

Severity (past week) of contamination obsessions and cleaning compulsions

1. *How much of your time is occupied by these obsessions and compulsions?*
   - 0 = **No time at all.**
   - 1 = **Rarely** present during the past week, often not on a daily basis, typically <3 hr/week.
   - 2 = **Occasionally, >3 hr/week, but <1 hr/day** – occasional intrusion, need to perform compulsions, or avoidance (occurs no >5 times a day).
   - 3 = **Frequently, 1 to 3 hr/day** – frequent intrusion, need to perform compulsions, or avoidance (occurs >8 times a day, but most hours of the day are free of these obsessions, compulsions, and related avoidance).
   - 4 = **Almost always, >3 and up to 8 hr/day** – very frequent intrusion, need to perform compulsions, or avoidance (occurs >8 times a day and occurs during most hours of the day).
   - 5 = **Always, >8 hr/day** – near constant intrusion of obsessions, need to perform compulsions, or avoidance (too numerous to count and an hour rarely passes without several obsessions, compulsions and/or avoidance).

2. *How much distress do these obsessions and related compulsions cause?*
   - 0 = **No distress.**
   - 1 = **Minimal,** when symptoms are present they are minimally distressing.
   - 2 = **Mild,** some clear distress present, but not too disturbing.
   - 3 = **Moderate,** disturbing, but still tolerable.
   - 4 = **Severe,** very disturbing.
   - 5 = **Extreme,** near constant and disabling distress.

3. *How much do these obsessions and related compulsions interfere with your family life, friendships, or ability to perform well at work or at school?*

   0 = **No interference**.

   1 = **Minimal**, slight interference with social or occupational activities, overall performance not impaired.

   2 = **Mild**, some interference with social or occupational activities, overall performance affected to a small degree.

   3 = **Moderate**, definite interference with social or occupational performance but still manageable.

   4 = **Severe interference**, causes substantial impairment in social or occupational performance.

   5 = **Extreme**, incapacitating interference.

Checklist of collecting and hoarding obsessions and compulsions

Checklist check once (✓) for any symptoms present during the past week.

This is a distinctive category that at times overlaps with concerns about doing harm. Check only if clear obsessions or compulsions that include collecting and hoarding are present.

Obsessions
___ Content involves needing to save things
___ Content involves distress over discarding things
___ Unable to decide to throw things away
___ Obsessions about losing things

Compulsions
___ Hoarding

___ Mental rituals that relate to hoarding

Avoidance
___ Intentional avoidance of places or things because of these obsessions or compulsions

Other symptoms in this category (describe):
_____
_____

Symptoms in this category were present during the past week?
   Yes   No
If yes, complete the next page. If no, skip to next section.

131

Severity (past week) of collecting and hoarding

1. *How much of your time is occupied by these obsessions and compulsions?*
   - 0 = **No time at all**.
   - 1 = **Rarely** present during the past week, often not on a daily basis, typically <3 hr/week.
   - 2 = **Occasionally, >3 hr/week, but <1 hr/day** – occasional intrusion, need to perform compulsions, or avoidance (occurs no >5 times a day).
   - 3 = **Frequently**, 1 to 3 hr/day – frequent intrusion, need to perform compulsions, or avoidance (occurs >8 times a day, but most hours of the day are free of these obsessions, compulsions, and related avoidance).
   - 4 = **Almost always, >3 and up to 8 hr/day** – very frequent intrusion, need to perform compulsions, or avoidance (occurs >8 times a day and occurs during most hours of the day).
   - 5 = **Always, >8 hr/day** – near constant intrusion of obsessions, need to perform compulsions, or avoidance (too numerous to count and an hour rarely passes without several obsessions, compulsions and/or avoidance).

2. *How much distress do these obsessions and related compulsions cause?*
   - 0 = **No distress**.
   - 1 = **Minimal**, when symptoms are present they are minimally distressing.
   - 2 = **Mild**, some clear distress present, but not too disturbing.
   - 3 = **Moderate**, disturbing, but still tolerable.
   - 4 = **Severe**, very disturbing.
   - 5 = **Extreme**, near constant and disabling distress.

3. *How much do these obsessions and related compulsions interfere with your family life, friendships, or ability to perform well at work or at school?*

0 = **No interference**.

1 = **Minimal**, slight interference with social or occupational activities, overall performance not impaired.

2 = **Mild**, some interference with social or occupational activities, overall performance affected to a small degree.

3 = **Moderate**, definite interference with social or occupational performance but still manageable.

4 = **Severe interference**, causes substantial impairment in social or occupational performance.

5 = **Extreme**, incapacitating interference.

Somatic obsessions and compulsions symptoms

Checklist check once (✓) for any other symptoms present during the past week.

Do not include symptoms related to body dysmorphic disorder or hypochondriasis. In hypochondriasis subjects believe that they have a serious illness or they are preoccupied with the idea that they do have a serious illness.

Somatic obsessions
___ Content involves illness or disease

Related compulsions
___ Checking or other compulsions related to somatic obsessions
___ Mental rituals other than checking related to somatic obsessions

Avoidance – somatic obsessions
___ Intentional avoidance of people, places or things because of any of the above obsessions or compulsions concerning illness or disease

Other symptoms in this category (describe):
_____
_____

Symptoms in this category were present during the past week?
Yes   No
If yes, complete the next page. If no, skip to next section.

Severity (past week) of somatic obsessions and compulsions*

1. *How much of your time is occupied by these obsessions and compulsions?*
   0 = **No time at all**.
   1 = **Rarely** present during the past week, often not on a daily basis, typically <3 hours/week.
   2 = **Occasionally, >3 hr/week, but <1 hr/day** – occasional intrusion, need to perform compulsions, or avoidance (occurs no >5 times a day).
   3 = **Frequently, 1 to 3 hr/day** – frequent intrusion, need to perform compulsions, or avoidance (occurs >8 times a day, but most hours of the day are free of these obsessions, compulsions, and related avoidance).
   4 = **Almost always, >3 and up to 8 hr/day** – very frequent intrusion, need to perform compulsions, or avoidance (occurs >8 times a day and occurs during most hours of the day).
   5 = **Always, >8 hr/day** – near constant intrusion of obsessions, need to perform compulsions, or avoidance (too numerous to count and an hour rarely passes without several obsessions, compulsions and/or avoidance).

2. *How much distress do these obsessions and related compulsions cause?*
   0 = **No distress**.
   1 = **Minimal**, when symptoms are present they are minimally distressing.
   2 = **Mild**, some clear distress present, but not too disturbing.
   3 = **Moderate**, disturbing, but still tolerable.
   4 = **Severe**, very disturbing.
   5 = **Extreme**, near constant and disabling distress.

3. *How much do these obsessions and related compulsions interfere with your family life, friendships, or ability to perform well at work or at school?*

0 = **No interference**.

1 = **Minimal**, slight interference with social or occupational activities, overall performance not impaired.

2 = **Mild**, some interference with social or occupational activities, overall performance affected to a small degree.

3 = **Moderate**, definite interference with social or occupational performance but still manageable.

4 = **Severe interference**, causes substantial impairment in social or occupational performance.

5 = **Extreme**, incapacitating interference.

Miscellaneous symptoms

Checklist check once (✓) for any other symptoms present during the past week.

Miscellaneous obsessions
___ Superstitious fears
___ Luck or unlucky numbers
___ Colours with special significance
___ Intrusive nonsense sounds, words or music
___ Intrusive (non-violent) images
___ Need to know or remember certain things

Compulsions
___ Superstitious behaviour
___ Related compulsions
___ Related compulsions
___ Related compulsions

___ Related compulsions
___ Excessive list making

___ Compulsions are: knowing, remembering
___ Obsessive slowness

Avoidance associated with miscellaneous obsessions and compulsions
___ Intentional avoidance of places or things because of these obsessions or compulsions

Other symptoms in this category (describe):

_____

_____

Symptoms in this category were present during the past week?
    Yes   No
If yes, complete the next page. If no, skip to next section.

Severity (past week) of miscellaneous obsessions and compulsions*

1. *How much of your time is occupied by these obsessions and compulsions?*
   - 0 = **No time at all.**
   - 1 = **Rarely** present during the past week, often not on a daily basis, typically <3 hr/week.
   - 2 = **Occasionally, >3 hr/week, but <1 hr/day** – occasional intrusion, need to perform compulsions, or avoidance (occurs no >5 times a day).
   - 3 = **Frequently, 1 to 3 hr/day** – frequent intrusion, need to perform compulsions, or avoidance (occurs >8 times a day, but most hours of the day are free of these obsessions, compulsions, and related avoidance).
   - 4 = **Almost always, >3 and up to 8 hr/day** – very frequent intrusion, need to perform compulsions, or avoidance (occurs >8 times a day and occurs during most hours of the day).
   - 5 = **Always, >8 hr/day** – near constant intrusion of obsessions, need to perform compulsions, or avoidance (too numerous to count and an hour rarely passes without several obsessions, compulsions and/or avoidance).

2. *How much distress do these obsessions and related compulsions cause?*
   - 0 = **No distress.**
   - 1 = **Minimal,** when symptoms are present they are minimally distressing.
   - 2 = **Mild,** some clear distress present, but not too disturbing.
   - 3 = **Moderate,** disturbing, but still tolerable.
   - 4 = **Severe,** very disturbing.
   - 5 = **Extreme,** near constant and disabling distress.

3. *How much do these obsessions and related compulsions interfere with your family life, friendships, or ability to perform well at work or at school?*

   0 = **No interference**.
   1 = **Minimal**, slight interference with social or occupational activities, overall performance not impaired.
   2 = **Mild**, some interference with social or occupational activities, overall performance affected to a small degree.
   3 = **Moderate**, definite interference with social or occupational performance but still manageable.
   4 = **Severe interference**, causes substantial impairment in social or occupational performance.
   5 = **Extreme**, incapacitating interference.

* Just include the obsessions and compulsions listed under 'Miscellaneous symptoms' in making these severity ratings.

Global obsessive-compulsive symptom severity

Indicate your best judgment concerning which symptom categories are present. Review with the patient how well their obsessions and compulsions fit within a given symptom category: 2 = clearly present and symptoms are readily understood in terms of a given symptom dimension; 1 = might be present, but significant uncertainty exists such that their symptoms are not readily understood in terms of a given symptom dimension; 0 = symptoms within a given dimension were absent or 'probably absent' during the past week.

_____ Aggressive obsessions and related compulsions
_____ Sexual and religious obsessions and related compulsions
_____ Symmetry, ordering, counting, and arranging obsessions and compulsions
_____ Contamination obsessions and cleaning compulsions
_____ Collecting and hoarding
_____ Somatic obsessions and compulsions
_____ Miscellaneous obsessions and compulsions

Rank order the symptom categories by severity for the past week. 1 = most severe, 2 = next most severe, and so on. Please mark each category. If symptoms were absent during the past week, place a '0' in the space provided.

_____ Aggressive obsessions and related compulsions
_____ Sexual and religious obsessions and related compulsions
_____ Symmetry, ordering, counting, and arranging obsessions and compulsions
_____ Contamination obsessions and cleaning compulsions
_____ Collecting and hoarding obsessions and compulsions
_____ Somatic obsessions and compulsions
_____ Miscellaneous obsessions and compulsions

List the patient's most prominent obsessive compulsive symptoms:

1. _____
2. _____
3. _____

What is the worst thing that the patient worries will happen if she/he did not respond to obsessive thoughts or urges to perform compulsions or rituals? Please describe:

_____

_____

How certain is the patient that this feared consequence is reasonable and will actually occur?

0 = Certain that the feared consequence will not happen
1 = Mostly certain that the feared consequence will not happen
2 = Unsure whether or not the feared consequence will or won't happen
3 = Mostly certain that that the feared consequence will happen
4 = Certain that the feared consequence will happen

Finally review all obsessive-compulsive symptoms endorsed as occurring during the past week (excluding 'other' symptoms judged not be bona fide obsessive-compulsive symptoms) and make a global severity rating for the past week using the ordinal scales on the next page and complete the score sheet.

Reliability of informant(s) Excellent = 0   Good = 1   Fair = 2   Poor = 3

Global severity obsessions and compulsions (past week)

1. *How much of your time is occupied by these obsessions and compulsions?*

   0 = **No time at all**.

   1 = **Rarely** present during the past week, often not on a daily basis, typically <3 hr/week.

   2 = **Occasionally, >3 hr/week, but <1 hr/day** – occasional intrusion, need to perform compulsions, or avoidance (occurs no >5 times a day).

   3 = **Frequently, 1 to 3 hr/day** – frequent intrusion, need to perform compulsions, or avoidance (occurs >8 times a day, but most hours of the day are free of these obsessions, compulsions, and related avoidance).

   4 = **Almost always, >3 and up to 8 hr/day** – very frequent intrusion, need to perform compulsions, or avoidance (occurs >8 times a day and occurs during most hours of the day).

   5 = **Always, >8 hr/day** – near constant intrusion of obsessions, need to perform compulsions, or avoidance (too numerous to count and an hour rarely passes without several obsessions, compulsions and/or avoidance).

2. *How much distress do these obsessions and related compulsions cause?*

   0 = **No distress**.

   1 = **Minimal**, when symptoms are present they are minimally distressing.

   2 = **Mild**, some clear distress present, but not too disturbing.

   3 = **Moderate**, disturbing, but still tolerable.

   4 = **Severe**, very disturbing.

   5 = **Extreme**, near constant and disabling distress.

3. *How much do these obsessions and related compulsions interfere with your family life, friendships, or ability to perform well at work or at school?*

0 = **No interference**.

1 = **Minimal**, slight interference with social or occupational activities, overall performance not impaired.

2 = **Mild**, some interference with social or occupational activities, overall performance affected to a small degree.

3 = **Moderate**, definite interference with social or occupational performance but still manageable.

4 = **Severe interference**, causes substantial impairment in social or occupational performance.

5 = **Extreme**, incapacitating interference.

DY-BOCS score sheet

Patient's name	Today's date: _/_/_
Clinician	mm dd yy

DY-BOCS clinician severity ratings by symptom category for the past week

Symptom category	Time (0–5)	Interference (0–5)	Distress (0–5)	Total (0–15)
Aggressive				
Sexual and religious				
Symmetry, ordering, counting and arranging				
Contamination and cleaning				
Hoarding and collecting				
Somatic				
Miscellaneous				

2. DY-DOCS global severity ratings for the past week

	Time (0–5)	Interference (0–5)	Distress (0–5)	Total (0–15)
All Obsessions and Compulsions				

Time required to complete the ratings _____ minutes

OC spectrum symptoms

Other somatic obsessions*

___ Content involves bodily appearance

___ Content involves food or eating

___ Content concerns the urge to pluck hair

___ Content concerns the urge to pick skin

Related compulsions

___ Related grooming compulsions

___ Related dressing compulsions

___ Related eating habits

___ Related compulsions related to physical exercise

___ Trichotillomania

___ Skin picking

Obsessions related to separation or union*

___ Concerns about being separated from a close family member

___ Concerns about becoming or being too much like another person

Compulsions

___ Compulsions to prevent the loss of a close family member

___ Related compulsions

Tic-related obsessions*

___ Staring rituals

___ Urge to repeat something you heard

* As in the original Y-BOCS, do not include these obsessions and compulsions in the severity ratings. Specialized rated instruments should be employed to rate separation anxiety disorder, tic disorders, eating disorders, body dysmorphic disorder, and trichotillomania. They are included here to document OC spectrum symptoms for research purposes.

Clinical Global Impression (CGI)

The Clinical Global Impression (CGI) is a brief 3-item clinician-rated scale that assesses illness severity, improvement/change, and response to treatment. The illness severity and improvement items are more frequently used by clinicians and researchers than the therapeutic response section, and for that reason only the former have been reproduced in this volume.

Reference
Guy, W. (1976). Early Clinical Drug Evaluation Program (ECDEU) *Assessment Manual for Psychopharmacology*. US Department of Health, Education and Welfare, Publication. **ADM 76–338**. Rockville, Md: National Institute of Mental Health, 217–222.

Clinical Global Impression Scale for Severity

The rating considers the clinician's entire experience with the disorder under investigation and the severity of that condition at the current time. Note that it is the severity of the particular condition that is rated, and not psychiatric illness generally.

Routine clinical CGI(s) differs from the CGI(s) scale usually used for research by 1 point.

Routine clinical CGI(s) is coded on a 0 to 6 scale as follows:	Research CGI(s) is coded on a 0 to 7 scale as follows:
0 = not ill	0 = not assessed
1 = borderline ill	1 = normal, not ill
2 = mildly ill	2 = borderline ill
3 = moderately ill	3 = mildly ill
4 = markedly ill	4 = moderately ill
5 = severely ill	5 = markedly ill
6 = among the most extremely ill	6 = severely ill
x = not assessed.	7 = among the most extremely ill

Clinical Global Impression Scale for Improvement

The rating considers the degree of change since the start of the current treatment plan. The rating does not consider whether the improvement is related to therapy or not.

Routine clinical CGI(i) is coded as follows:	Research CGI(i) is coded as follows:
+3 = very much improved	0 = not assesed
+2 = much improved	1 = very much improved
+1 = minimally improved	2 = much improved
0 = unchanged	3 = minimally improved
−1 = minimally worse	4 = unchanged
−2 = much worse	5 = minimally worse
−3 = very much worse	6 = much worse
x = not assessed	7 = very much worse

The CGI is available in the public domain.

Index